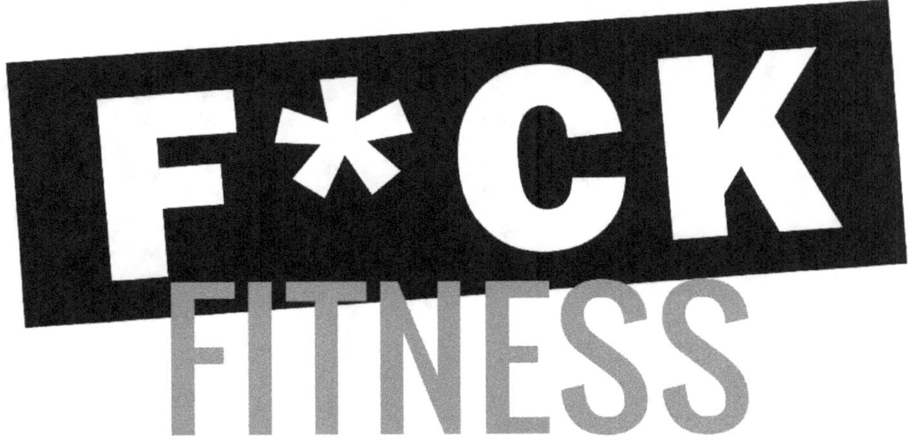

The Badass Guide to Smashing Fitness Culture One F*cking Rep at a Time!

Logan West

Table Of Contents

Why Skipping the Gym Doesn't Make You a Failure

Welcome to the book that fitness culture doesn't want you to read. If you've ever skipped the gym, eaten carbs without regret, or looked at a "motivational" workout quote and thought, "Fuck that," then congratulations—you're exactly where you need to be. This book isn't here to guilt you into burpees or make you feel bad for preferring a Netflix binge over a spin class. It's here to blow up all the bullshit that fitness culture has been feeding you and help you embrace a life that actually makes you happy.

Let's get one thing straight right off the bat: skipping the gym doesn't make you a failure. Seriously. You're not a garbage human being because you didn't wake up at 5 a.m. to run five miles or because you'd rather eat a donut than a protein bar that tastes like chalk. Fitness culture would have you believe that if you're not drenched in sweat and chugging a green smoothie, you're doing life wrong. But guess what? Fitness culture is full of shit.

Here's the truth: you don't owe anyone a "perfect" body or a daily step count. You don't have to turn your life into a series of workouts, macros, and guilt-ridden cheat meals. And you sure as hell don't need to listen to Karen from accounting tell you how she burned 500 calories before breakfast. This book is about flipping the middle finger to all of that and figuring out what works for *you.*

Maybe you've been stuck in the cycle of gym memberships you never use, fitness gadgets that gather dust, and workout routines that make you want to cry. Or maybe you've been guilted into believing that you're less-than because you don't fit the mold of what fitness "should" look like. Well, fuck that noise. This book is here to help you break free from the rules, the guilt, and the pressure, and to remind you that your worth has absolutely nothing to do with how many squats you did today.

We'll tackle the lies the fitness industry loves to sell you (spoiler: carbs are not your enemy), explore why "beach body" is the dumbest phrase ever invented, and give you tools to tell the fitness police to fuck right off. Whether you want to move your body, rest it, or just eat a pizza in peace, you'll find permission to do it here—with zero guilt and a whole lot of sass.

So, if you're ready to embrace body positivity, laugh at fitness fails, and build a relationship with movement that doesn't suck the joy out of your life, then grab a snack, get comfortable, and let's dive in. This isn't about sweating harder or eating cleaner—it's about living unapologetically. Welcome to *Fck* Fitness.* Let's get started.

Chapter 1

The Fitness Myth: How We Got Brainwashed Into Thinking We Need to Sweat to Be Worthy

The History of Fitness Bullshit: How Fitness Culture Convinced Us We're Never Good Enough

Let's get one thing clear: fitness culture didn't always exist. Our ancestors weren't doing CrossFit in caves or signing up for Spartan Races to prove their worth. They were just out there trying to survive, hunting mammoths and gathering berries without worrying about whether their ass looked good in leggings. Somewhere along the way, though, shit went sideways. We went from just living to constantly chasing some unattainable standard of "fitness," and now we're all stuck in this ridiculous hamster wheel of self-loathing and overpriced gym memberships.

So how did we get here? Let me introduce you to the birth of fitness culture—the unholy love child of capitalism, societal pressures, and the collective human desire to look hot naked. Back in the day, fitness wasn't about aesthetics; it was about function. People worked hard because they had to, not because they wanted to fit into skinny jeans.

But then along came the Industrial Revolution, and suddenly, we weren't plowing fields or running from predators anymore. We were sitting at desks, getting soft, and freaking the fuck out about it.

Enter the snake oil salesmen of the early fitness industry. These assholes saw an opportunity and ran with it. They started marketing bullshit like vibrating belts that promised to jiggle the fat off your ass and "health tonics" that were probably just sugar water. And the people? Oh, they ate that shit up. Because if there's one thing humanity loves, it's an easy fix that doesn't actually work.

Fast forward to the 20th century, and things got even worse. The rise of Hollywood brought with it the first wave of body image obsession. Suddenly, everyone wanted to look like the stars on the big screen, even though those stars were starving themselves and popping diet pills like candy. Fitness wasn't about health anymore; it was about vanity. And the fitness industry? Well, they saw dollar signs.

Gyms started popping up everywhere, promising to turn you into a Greek god if you just forked over your hard-earned cash. And if you didn't? Well, clearly, you were a lazy piece of shit who didn't care about yourself. The messaging was clear: if you weren't sweating your ass off in a gym, you were failing at life. And we bought it. We bought it hard.

By the time the 80s rolled around, fitness culture was in full fucking swing. This was the era of aerobics, jazzercise, and Richard Simmons telling you to "sweat to the oldies." Let's not forget the spandex-clad monsters like Jane Fonda, who made us believe that bouncing around in leg warmers was the key to happiness. It didn't matter if you hated every second of it; what mattered was that you looked good while doing it.

The 90s took it up a notch with the rise of gym culture. Suddenly, everyone had to have a membership to some big-box fitness chain with shiny machines and mirrors on every surface. It wasn't just about working out—it was about being seen working out. If you didn't post up at the squat rack or flex in the mirror, did you even lift, bro?

Then came the 2000s, and with it, the rise of "wellness." Fitness culture slapped on a mask of self-care and started calling itself "holistic." But don't be fooled—it was the same old bullshit, just repackaged. Instead of just working out, now you had to drink green juice, meditate, and do yoga on a $200 mat while wearing $100 leggings. And if you weren't doing it all, well, clearly, you didn't love yourself enough.

And let's not even get started on the social media era. Instagram became the breeding ground for fitness influencers selling you detox teas, booty band workouts, and the idea that you're only worthy if you look like a filtered version of yourself. Every scroll is a slap in the face, reminding you that you're not doing enough, sweating enough, or looking hot enough.

Here's the thing: fitness culture thrives on making you feel like shit. If you feel good about yourself, you won't buy their products, sign up for their classes, or spend your rent money on a Peloton bike. So they keep moving the goalposts. Six-pack abs? Not enough. Now you need a peach-shaped ass, toned arms, and the ability to run a marathon without breaking a sweat. It's a never-ending cycle of "not enough," and it's designed to keep you hooked.

But here's the dirty little secret they don't want you to know: fitness isn't a one-size-fits-all thing. You don't have to sweat your ass off in a gym or count every calorie to be healthy. You don't have to punish yourself for enjoying food or feel guilty for skipping a workout. And you sure as fuck don't have to compare yourself to some airbrushed influencer who probably doesn't even look like that in real life.

The truth is, fitness culture has been lying to you your whole life. It's time to call bullshit on the whole damn thing. You are not a failure because you don't fit their mold. You are not lazy because you'd rather nap than do burpees. And you are not unworthy because you don't have a six-pack.

Fitness isn't about looking a certain way or proving your worth through sweat. It's about moving your body in a way that feels good, eating food that makes you happy, and living a life that brings you joy. It's about finding what works for you, not what some asshole on Instagram says you should be doing.

So fuck the fitness myths, fuck the pressure to conform, and fuck anyone who tries to tell you that you're not enough. You are enough, exactly as you are. And if the fitness industry doesn't like that? Well, they can kiss your unapologetic, happy-ass goodbye.

Sweat Worship: Why People Treat Working Out Like a Religion and Why You Don't Have To

Let's talk about the cult of sweat worship. You know the one. It's the religion where the altar is a treadmill, the holy water is protein shakes, and the high priests are Instagram influencers screaming about "no excuses" and "beast mode." Their gospel? Sweat more, suffer harder, and maybe, just maybe, you'll be worthy of self-love. Sound familiar? Of course, it does—because fitness culture has convinced us that working out is the ultimate path to redemption, and if you're not drenched in sweat by 7 a.m., you're failing at life.

But here's the truth they don't want you to know: you don't have to worship at the church of sweat to be happy, healthy, or worthy. Working out isn't a moral obligation, and it sure as fuck doesn't determine your value as a human being. So why the hell do so many people treat it like it does?

It all starts with the messaging. Somewhere along the line, society decided that sweat equals virtue. If you're sweating, you're grinding. You're hustling. You're proving your dedication to becoming a "better" version of yourself. Never mind that half the time, you're just dripping in sweat because it's 90 degrees outside, and you accidentally wore a gray T-shirt. Sweat has been marketed as the ultimate symbol of effort, and effort has become synonymous with self-worth.

And then there are the slogans. You've seen them plastered on gym walls and emblazoned on tank tops: "Sweat is fat crying." "No pain, no gain." "Pain is weakness leaving the body." Bullshit, bullshit, and more bullshit. Sweat isn't fat crying—it's your body trying not to overheat. Pain isn't weakness leaving the body—it's your muscles screaming, "What the actual fuck are you doing to me?" And if you're drenched in sweat but still hating every second of your workout, what exactly are you gaining?

Let's not forget the people who treat their workouts like a goddamn spiritual experience. You know the type. They post sweaty selfies with captions like, "Church of the Iron today 🙏" or "My workout is my therapy." And hey, if that's genuinely what works for them, good for them. But here's the thing: you don't have to find enlightenment through deadlifts. You don't have to pretend that sweating your ass off on a stationary bike is some kind of transcendental journey.

Sweat worship also thrives on guilt. Didn't work out today? Cue the inner voice that says, "Wow, you're really letting yourself go, huh?" Didn't burn enough calories? "Better skip dinner, fatty." It's relentless, and it's toxic as hell. The fitness industry loves guilt because it keeps you coming back for more. Feel bad about skipping a workout? Sign up for another boot camp. Feel guilty about eating a donut? Hit the gym for an extra hour. It's a vicious cycle, and sweat is the currency that fuels it.

But let's get real for a second: not everyone enjoys working out. And that's okay. The fitness industry wants you to believe that if you're not grinning through a grueling workout, you're doing it wrong. But the truth is, sweating isn't supposed to be a fucking carnival. You don't have to love burpees, adore spin class, or find joy in lifting heavy things and putting them back down. You're allowed to think that shit sucks.

The problem with sweat worship is that it turns exercise into a performance. It's not enough to just move your body; you have to move it in a way that's visible, intense, and Instagram-worthy. You can't just go for a walk—you have to track your steps and share your stats. You can't just stretch—you have to post a time-lapse of your yoga flow with inspirational music. Fitness culture has turned working out into a spectator sport, and honestly, it's exhausting.

And can we talk about the obsession with "earning" your food through sweat? This one really grinds my gears. You don't have to do a single goddamn squat to deserve a slice of pizza. You don't have to burn 500 calories to justify eating a cupcake. Food is not a reward, and sweat is not a currency. You're allowed to eat what you want, when you want, without treating it like a transaction.

Here's the thing: your worth isn't measured by how much you sweat, how many calories you burn, or how many reps you can crank out. Sweat worship would have you believe otherwise, but it's all a load of crap. You don't have to prove your dedication to the cult of fitness by torturing yourself in the gym. You don't have to buy into the idea that suffering equals success.

Instead, let's reframe what movement means. It doesn't have to involve sweat at all. Maybe for you, it's dancing in your kitchen to '80s hits, strolling through the park, or stretching on the floor while binge-watching your favorite show. Movement is supposed to feel good—not like a punishment for existing.

If sweating makes you happy, then by all means, sweat your heart out. But if you're forcing yourself to suffer through workouts you hate just because you think you're supposed to, it's time to rethink the whole damn thing. Movement doesn't have to be about sweat, effort, or proving anything to anyone. It's about finding what works for you and doing it on your terms.

So the next time someone tries to guilt you into a workout you don't want to do, just smile and say, "Thanks, but no thanks. I've got better shit to do." Whether that's napping, eating carbs, or finding a form of movement that doesn't make you miserable, you're already winning. Because you don't owe anyone sweat. You owe yourself happiness. And that's the kind of worship that actually matters.

"Fitness Culture is Like a Cult, but Instead of Kool-Aid, They Make You Drink Protein Shakes"

Fitness culture is, without a doubt, one of the most bizarre cults of modern life. You've got the rituals (morning workouts), the sacred texts (meal plans and macros), the hierarchy (trainers, influencers, and that one guy who never skips leg day), and, of course, the overpriced, questionable beverages (protein shakes that taste like wet cardboard). The only thing missing is a charismatic leader in a tracksuit promising enlightenment through squats. But don't worry—there are plenty of wannabe leaders out there, armed with hashtags and unsolicited advice.

Let's break this shit down, shall we?

First, there's the initiation ritual. When you join the cult of fitness culture, you're immediately bombarded with jargon: reps, sets, macros, HIIT, and, of course, the infamous "clean eating." It's like learning a new fucking language. If you don't know what a burpee is, or if you confuse a deadlift with some kind of goth dance move, you're already an outsider. But don't worry—the cult will gladly take your money to teach you the lingo.

Once you're initiated, it's time to prove your devotion. Like any cult worth its salt, fitness culture demands loyalty. You can't just show up once or twice a week—you have to make it your entire fucking personality. Post your sweaty selfies, hashtag your workouts, and tell anyone who'll listen about your new "journey." Bonus points if you buy the matching gym outfit and drink the protein shake they're all hawking. If you're not repping the brand, are you even trying?

Now, let's talk about the Kool-Aid—except in this cult, it's protein shakes, green juices, and pre-workout powder that looks suspiciously like cocaine. These concoctions are marketed as the key to your success, promising everything from muscle gains to fat loss to eternal happiness. But let's be real—most of them taste like shit. I mean, if chalk and grass had a baby, it would taste better than half the shit being sold at supplement stores. But hey, it's all part of the ritual. If you're not choking down something disgusting, are you even committed?

Then there's the dogma. Every cult needs rules, and fitness culture is no exception. Rule #1: Thou shalt not eat carbs. Rule #2: Thou shalt sacrifice thy weekends for meal prep. Rule #3: Thou shalt worship the almighty protein. If you break the rules, expect a barrage of guilt and judgment, either from yourself or from the self-appointed prophets in your life. You know the type—Karen from accounting who won't shut up about her keto diet, or Brad at the gym who thinks intermittent fasting is the secret to life.

And don't get me started on the sacred gatherings, aka group fitness classes. These are basically cult meetings with better lighting and worse music. Everyone's wearing the same overpriced leggings, sweating to the same shitty playlist, and pretending they're not silently competing with each other. If you've ever been to a spin class, you know what I'm talking about. It's 45 minutes of pain, shouting, and inspirational bullshit like, "Push harder—your future self will thank you!" Yeah, my future self is gonna thank me when I order pizza after this.

Of course, every cult needs a hierarchy, and fitness culture is no different. At the top, you've got the influencers—those impossibly fit, annoyingly photogenic people who make money by convincing you that you, too, can look like them if you buy their e-book and detox tea.

Below them are the trainers, the ones who simultaneously motivate you and make you question every life choice that led you to a 5 a.m. boot camp. And at the bottom? Us regular folks, sweating our asses off and wondering why we thought this was a good idea.

But perhaps the most cult-like aspect of fitness culture is the promise of salvation. They tell you that if you just work hard enough, suffer long enough, and buy enough of their shit, you'll achieve the ultimate reward: the "perfect" body. It's the fitness version of heaven, and it's just as unattainable. No matter how much you sweat, no matter how many protein shakes you choke down, it's never enough. There's always something else to improve, always another goal to chase. It's a treadmill you can never get off—literally and figuratively.

And let's not forget the excommunication process. If you dare to leave the cult—if you stop going to the gym, quit your meal plan, or admit that you don't give a fuck about your abs—expect to be judged. The fitness police will swoop in, armed with unsolicited advice and condescending comments. "Oh, you're not working out anymore? That's fine, as long as you're happy." Bitch, I *am* happy. Happier than you, probably, because I'm not spending half my paycheck on supplements and sweat-wicking socks.

But here's the thing: you don't have to drink the Kool-Aid—or the protein shake—to be healthy or happy. You don't have to join the cult, follow their rules, or buy into their bullshit. Fitness doesn't have to be a religion, and you don't have to worship at the altar of sweat.

If you love working out, great. If you hate it, also great. You're not a better person because you crushed a spin class, and you're not a worse person because you skipped leg day. Fitness culture wants you to believe that your worth is tied to your workouts, but that's just another lie they're selling.

So the next time someone tries to recruit you into the cult, just smile and say, "No thanks—I'm good." Then go home, eat some carbs, and do something that actually makes you happy. Because life is too short to drink shitty protein shakes and pretend to enjoy burpees. Fuck the cult. Be your own damn guru.

Chapter 2

"Beach Body" BS: Why Society's Definition of Fitness Can Go Fuck Itself

The Myth of the Perfect Body: Spoiler: It's Unattainable and Subjective as Fuck

Let's just rip the Band-Aid off right now: the "perfect body" is a myth. A scam. A colossal pile of steaming bullshit invented by marketing execs, fashion magazines, and gym bros who think grunting loudly makes them more impressive. The idea that there's one specific body type that's the gold standard of beauty, health, and worth? Yeah, that's about as real as the Easter Bunny. And yet, society has been shoving this unattainable ideal down our throats for decades, making us feel like trash for not fitting into its narrow, arbitrary mold.

First off, let's talk about what society considers a "perfect" body. For women, it's usually some combination of flat stomach, perky boobs, a Kardashian-esque ass, and legs for days—but not too muscular, because *heaven forbid* you look "manly." For men, it's all about broad shoulders, chiseled abs, and biceps that look like they could crush a watermelon.

Basically, society wants us all to look like action figures or airbrushed Instagram models, and anything less is deemed unworthy.

Here's the kicker, though: this so-called perfect body is completely subjective. What's considered ideal changes depending on the decade, the culture, and whoever's currently in charge of the media. In the '50s, Marilyn Monroe's curves were the pinnacle of beauty. By the '90s, it was all about being waif-thin like Kate Moss. Now, it's somewhere between "slim thick" and "muscle Barbie," depending on who you ask. It's like trying to hit a moving target while blindfolded—it's fucking impossible.

And even if you *could* achieve this ever-changing ideal, it still wouldn't be enough. That's the dirty little secret of the fitness and beauty industries: they're designed to keep you chasing. Because if you ever actually felt good about yourself, you wouldn't buy their shit. Why do you think there's a new "must-have" product, workout trend, or diet every five minutes? They thrive on your insecurities, and they'll do whatever it takes to keep them alive and well.

But let's get real for a second. The idea of a perfect body isn't just unattainable—it's harmful as fuck. It makes you scrutinize every inch of yourself in the mirror, obsess over numbers on a scale, and feel like a failure for having the audacity to exist in a body that doesn't look like it belongs on the cover of *Men's Health* or *Cosmopolitan.* It convinces you that your worth is tied to your appearance, and that's not just bullshit— it's dangerous.

Take a moment to think about all the time, money, and energy you've spent trying to achieve the "perfect" body. How many hours have you wasted sweating your ass off in workouts you hate, skipping meals, or

Googling things like "how to get rid of belly fat fast"? And for what? So you can post a thirst trap on Instagram and hope Karen from high school comments, "You look amazing, babe"? Fuck that noise.

And while we're on the subject, let's talk about the phrase "beach body." You've heard it a million times: "Get your beach body ready!" "Summer's coming—time to tone up!" As if the ocean gives a single flying fuck what you look like in a swimsuit. Spoiler alert: it doesn't. You don't need six-pack abs to lie on the sand or splash in the waves. You don't need a thigh gap to rock a bikini or a Speedo. If you have a body and you're at the beach, congratulations—you have a beach body. End of fucking story.

Of course, the fitness industry would have you believe otherwise. They've built an entire empire on the idea that you're not "beach ready" unless you've sculpted your body into some magazine-approved shape. It's all about selling you the dream: the abs, the tan, the confidence. But here's the thing they don't tell you: even the people in those ads don't look like that in real life. It's all lighting, angles, Photoshop, and a shit-ton of dehydration.

The "perfect body" myth also ignores the fact that bodies are supposed to be different. People come in all shapes, sizes, and configurations, and that's what makes the world interesting. Imagine how boring it would be if we all looked the same, like some dystopian army of gym mannequins. Diversity isn't just beautiful—it's fucking essential.

But society doesn't want you to celebrate your unique body. It wants you to feel bad about it so you'll spend your hard-earned cash trying to change it. And the fucked-up part is, even if you achieve your so-called "dream body," they'll find something else for you to fix. Your stomach's flat, but what about your arms? Your ass is toned, but what about your cellulite? It's a never-ending cycle of bullshit, and the only way to win is to stop playing the game.

So what's the alternative? How do you break free from the myth of the perfect body and start loving the one you're in? For starters, stop giving a fuck about what society says you should look like. Their standards are arbitrary, unrealistic, and rooted in greed. Your body is yours, and it's already worthy of love, respect, and a cute-ass swimsuit.

Next, start focusing on what your body can do, not just how it looks. Maybe it's carrying you through tough days, dancing like a maniac at weddings, or walking your dog every morning. Your body is fucking amazing, and it deserves credit for more than just fitting into a size whatever.

And finally, surround yourself with people and media that celebrate real bodies, not airbrushed fantasies. Unfollow the influencers who make you feel like shit and follow the ones who keep it real. Watch shows and movies with diverse casts that reflect the beauty of all body types. Remind yourself every damn day that you are enough, exactly as you are.

The myth of the perfect body is just that—a myth. It's unattainable, subjective, and a complete waste of your time and energy. So fuck it. Wear the bikini, eat the carbs, skip the workout, and live your life. Because you don't need society's approval to be happy, healthy, or fucking fabulous. You're already perfect, just as you are.

Beach Body Marketing Lies: Why the Phrase "Beach Body" Is Designed to Make You Feel Like Crap

Let's get real for a second: the phrase "beach body" is one of the most manipulative, guilt-inducing, and downright toxic pieces of marketing bullshit ever invented. The second someone utters those two words, you're instantly hit with a mental checklist of things you apparently need to fix before you're deemed worthy of stepping foot on sand. Flat stomach? Check. Zero cellulite? Check. Toned arms, thigh gap, and glowing skin? Double fucking check. It's like an unpaid internship for your self-esteem, and no one signed up for this shit.

Here's the truth: "beach body" is a weapon. It's a phrase created by the fitness and beauty industries to make you feel like crap about your natural, amazing, capable body so they can sell you shit you don't need. Gym memberships, detox teas, miracle creams, weight-loss apps, tanning oils, plastic surgery consultations—you name it, they're shoving it down your throat. Why? Because the more insecure you are, the more money you're willing to throw at the problem they've convinced you exists.

Let's rewind a bit and dissect what the term "beach body" even means. Spoiler alert: it doesn't mean jack shit. It's a completely made-up concept, as arbitrary as deciding that only people with purple hair can go to the beach. It's a way of gatekeeping enjoyment and relaxation, as if the ocean sent out a fucking memo declaring, "No abs, no entry."

The whole thing is especially ridiculous when you think about the actual purpose of the beach: to relax, soak up some sun, and maybe get sand in places you didn't think possible. The ocean doesn't give a fuck what you look like. The sand isn't judging your stretch marks. The seagulls definitely don't care if your thighs jiggle when you walk. And yet, we've been brainwashed into believing that the beach is some sort of exclusive runway where only the "perfect" are allowed to strut their shit.

Beach body marketing thrives on this insecurity. It pops up like clockwork every spring, bombarding you with ads that say, "Summer's coming! Are you ready?" Ready for what, exactly? To wear a swimsuit? To sit in a lounge chair? To eat a hot dog at a barbecue? It's not the goddamn Olympics. You don't need to train for it. And yet, they make it sound like you're failing at life if you're not hitting the gym six days a week and eating salad for every meal.

One of the sneakiest lies beach body marketing sells is the idea that there's a "deadline" for getting your body "ready." It's like they've decided summer is a performance, and you're the lead actor in a play no one asked to see. The idea that you're supposed to transform yourself in a matter of weeks—shedding pounds, toning muscles, and achieving the impossible—is pure, unadulterated bullshit.

And let's talk about the phrase "getting in shape." What shape are we even talking about here? A triangle? A rhombus? The insinuation is clear: whatever shape you're currently in isn't good enough. The whole thing is designed to make you feel like shit so you'll panic-buy a gym membership or the latest miracle diet plan. And guess what? None of it works long-term because the problem isn't your body—it's the unrealistic standards they're shoving down your throat.

Another hallmark of beach body marketing is the incessant focus on before-and-after photos. These gems are designed to convince you that you, too, can go from sad blob to toned goddess if you just follow their program. But let's get real for a second: those "before" pictures are often staged to look as unflattering as possible, while the "after" photos involve better lighting, strategic posing, and sometimes a healthy dose of Photoshop. It's smoke and mirrors, people, and it's designed to fuck with your head.

And can we please address the irony of calling it a "beach body"? The beach is literally one of the most casual, come-as-you-are places on earth. It's not a gala. It's not a black-tie event. It's a place where people eat greasy boardwalk fries, get sunburned, and accidentally flash strangers when a rogue wave hits. The idea that you need to look flawless for this is laughable.

But the fitness and beauty industries aren't laughing. They're raking in billions by convincing you that your natural, functional, incredible body is a "problem" that needs to be fixed. And it's not just about selling you products—it's about selling you shame. Every ad, every Instagram post, every influencer with a flat stomach and a bikini captioned "hard work pays off" is designed to make you feel like you're not enough.

Here's the thing: you are enough. Right now. As you are. Your body doesn't need a makeover to deserve the sun on your skin or the sand between your toes. You don't need abs to enjoy the ocean, and you sure as fuck don't need someone else's approval to wear a swimsuit.

Let's rewrite the rules. A "beach body" is any body that shows up at the beach. That's it. No detoxes, no boot camps, no crash diets required. Your stretch marks? Beautiful. Your belly rolls? Perfectly normal. Your cellulite? Literally just fat pushing through connective tissue—it's not a fucking crime scene.

The next time someone tries to sell you the idea that you need to "get ready" for summer, tell them to fuck right off. Summer isn't a contest, and your body isn't a project. It's the vessel that carries you through this messy, beautiful life, and it deserves respect—not shame.

So wear the swimsuit, eat the ice cream, and show up at the beach like the badass you are. Because the only thing you need to be "beach ready" is the audacity to exist. And you, my friend, are already perfect.

"Newsflash: If You Have a Body and You're at the Beach, You Have a Fucking Beach Body"

Here's the thing about "beach body" culture: it's built on the absolutely ridiculous premise that you need to look a certain way to hang out near sand and water. Let me break it down for you—if you have a body, and you're at the beach, congratulations, you've already achieved peak beach body status. There's no secret handshake, no membership card, and definitely no scale involved. You're there. You did it. Mission fucking accomplished.

Let me tell you about the first time I realized this earth-shattering truth. I was at the beach with a group of friends, all of us hauling coolers, towels, and an absurd amount of snacks. As we set up camp near the water, I noticed a guy nearby—probably mid-50s, wearing a pair of neon green swim trunks that should've come with a warning label. He had a glorious beer belly that defied gravity and a confidence that could rival Beyoncé's. He strutted down to the water, belly leading the way, and dove in like a majestic sea lion.

It was in that moment I had an epiphany: this man didn't give a single fuck. He wasn't worried about his abs (or lack thereof). He wasn't sucking in his gut or wondering if anyone was judging his stretch marks. He was just living his best goddamn life. And you know what? That's the energy we should all be channeling.

Compare that to the time I spent an entire vacation stressing over my "beach body." I'd gone on some ridiculous crash diet beforehand, sweating my ass off in workouts I hated and eating salads so sad they deserved a funeral. The result? I still felt insecure the entire time. Every time I sat down, I'd throw a towel over my stomach like some kind of makeshift invisibility cloak. God forbid anyone see me sitting like a normal human being with rolls because, apparently, that's a fucking crime.

Meanwhile, everyone else at the beach was just...existing. There were kids building sandcastles, parents chasing toddlers, and retirees playing bocce ball like it was the goddamn Olympics. Not a single person gave a shit about my stomach or my cellulite. Turns out, the only person judging me was me. And honestly, what a waste of energy.

One of my favorite beach moments happened a few years ago when I went on a family trip. My aunt, who gives absolutely zero fucks about societal expectations, decided to wear a bikini for the first time in decades. "If I wait until I lose 20 pounds, I'll never wear one," she declared while tying the strings of her top. And you know what? She rocked it. She lounged in her beach chair, sipping a margarita, and confidently called out to the waiter to bring her another. "Life's too short for ugly swimsuits," she said, and honestly, she's my hero.

Then there was the time I saw a group of older women at the beach who were clearly living their best lives. They had matching floppy hats, an arsenal of snacks, and zero fucks to give about what anyone thought.

One of them, who was easily in her 70s, got up and did a cartwheel—right there on the sand. Was it graceful? Hell no. Did she nail it? Also no. But the joy on her face was unmatched. She wasn't worried about whether her thighs jiggled or if she'd sandpapered her legs beforehand. She was just having fun, and it was fucking glorious.

Meanwhile, here we are, obsessing over whether our swimsuit covers enough or wondering if our tan lines are even. Why? Who decided the beach was a beauty pageant? Newsflash: it's not. The only judges are the seagulls, and they're too busy trying to steal your chips to give a shit about what you look like.

Let's also take a moment to talk about kids. Have you ever seen a child at the beach worrying about their body? Of course not. They're too busy digging holes, jumping waves, and eating sandy popsicles. Kids don't give a fuck about beach bodies. They care about having a good time. Somewhere along the way, we lose that carefree attitude, and instead of enjoying the beach, we start treating it like a stage where we have to perform.

One summer, I went on a trip with a friend who'd just had a baby. She was nervous about wearing a swimsuit because, in her words, "everything's not where it used to be." But when we got to the beach, her baby had other plans. He immediately started flailing around, kicking sand everywhere and demanding to be carried into the water. Within minutes, she was laughing, splashing, and completely forgetting about her insecurities. Watching her have that much fun was a reminder that no one gives a fuck about your so-called imperfections when you're busy enjoying yourself.

And that's the secret to a true "beach body": it's not about how you look—it's about how you feel. If you're happy, comfortable, and having a good time, you've already won. Fuck the societal standards, the marketing lies, and the voice in your head telling you you're not good enough. You are. Right now. As you are.

So, the next time you're at the beach, channel your inner beer-belly guy, badass aunt, or carefree kid. Wear the swimsuit that makes you feel amazing, eat the snacks you love, and dive into the waves like you own the place. Because you do. And anyone who doesn't like it can fuck right off.

Chapter 3

Carbs Are Not the Enemy: Debunking the Fitness Industry's Favorite Lies

Carbs Are Fuel, Not Satan: Why Bread, Pasta, and Potatoes Are Your Friends

Let me make one thing crystal fucking clear right off the bat: carbs are not your enemy. Carbs are not the devil reincarnated into baguettes and spaghetti. Carbs are not out to ruin your life or sabotage your waistline. Carbs are fuel. They are delicious, versatile, life-giving little bundles of energy, and they deserve more respect than they've been getting from fitness culture.

So why the fuck did carbs get such a bad rap? Somewhere along the way, the fitness industry decided that bread, pasta, and potatoes were public enemy number one. "Cut out carbs," they said. "They make you fat," they said. What they didn't say was that this entire narrative is based on pseudoscience, marketing gimmicks, and the collective hatred of joy. Because let's face it: what is life without carbs?

The war on carbs probably started with some diet guru who decided to demonize them to sell a book. You know the type—the kind of person who thinks butter in coffee is a good idea and claims you can eat bacon for every meal as long as you avoid bread. These assholes made carbs the scapegoat for everything from weight gain to world hunger, and people bought it. Literally. Low-carb diets like Atkins and keto became the holy grail for anyone trying to shed a few pounds, and carbs got relegated to the "do not eat" list along with trans fats and cyanide.

But here's the thing: your body *needs* carbs. Carbs are your body's primary source of energy. When you eat carbs, your body breaks them down into glucose, which fuels everything from your brain to your muscles. Without carbs, you're basically running on fumes, and your body starts to freak the fuck out. That's why people on low-carb diets are always cranky as hell. They're not better than you—they're just hangry.

Let's talk about bread for a second. Bread is one of the oldest, most universal foods on the planet. Civilizations were literally built on bread. The pyramids didn't get built on kale and protein powder, my friend— they got built on bread. And yet, somehow, fitness culture decided that bread is evil. It's not. Bread is comforting, delicious, and full of nutrients if you're not buying the kind that feels like chewing on a sponge.

And then there's pasta, the MVP of comfort food. There's a reason why your first instinct after a shitty day is to make a big-ass bowl of spaghetti or dive face-first into a plate of mac and cheese. Pasta is like a hug for your soul, and anyone who says otherwise is a liar. Sure, the fitness industry will tell you to replace your pasta with zucchini noodles or spaghetti squash, but you and I both know that shit is not the same. It's a sad, watery imposter, and it will never bring you the joy that real pasta can.

Potatoes might be the most versatile carb of all. Fried, mashed, roasted, baked—potatoes are the backbone of comfort food. They've been feeding the masses for centuries, and yet, fitness culture treats them like a ticking time bomb of calories and carbs. "Skip the fries," they say. "Order a side salad instead." Fuck that. Order the fries. Life's too short to deny yourself the simple pleasure of crispy, golden perfection.

Fitness culture also loves to scare you with buzzwords like "high glycemic index" and "insulin spikes" when it comes to carbs. They'll tell you that eating a piece of bread is basically the same as injecting pure sugar into your veins. Spoiler alert: it's not. Your body knows how to handle carbs. It's literally designed to process them and turn them into energy. Unless you're diabetic or have a medical condition that requires you to monitor your blood sugar, you don't need to stress about this shit.

Another favorite lie is that carbs make you gain weight. Here's the truth: eating more calories than your body needs makes you gain weight. It doesn't matter if those calories come from carbs, fat, or protein. Blaming carbs for weight gain is like blaming your shoes for making you late—it's ignoring the bigger picture.

Let's not forget the fitness industry's obsession with "good" carbs versus "bad" carbs. Whole grains? Good. White bread? Bad. Sweet potatoes? Good. French fries? Bad. But here's the thing: labeling food as "good" or "bad" is a slippery slope that leads to food guilt and a fucked-up relationship with eating. You're not a better person because you chose quinoa over rice, and you're not a failure because you ate a donut. Food is food. Some of it's more nutritious than others, but none of it makes you a bad person.

Carbs also get a bad rap because they're delicious, and anything that tastes good is apparently suspicious in the world of fitness. Bread is fluffy. Pasta is creamy. Potatoes are crispy. Carbs bring joy, and fitness culture doesn't know what to do with that. They'd rather you chew on a piece of grilled chicken and pretend it's satisfying. Spoiler alert: it's not.

But the real kicker is how carbs are vilified for being "empty calories," as if every bite of food needs to justify its existence with a laundry list of nutrients. Sometimes, food is just supposed to taste good and make you happy. A warm bagel with cream cheese doesn't need to be a superfood—it just needs to be fucking delicious.

The bottom line? Carbs are not the enemy. Bread, pasta, potatoes, and all their carb-loaded friends are here to fuel your body, bring you joy, and make life a little more delicious. So the next time someone tries to convince you to skip the bread basket or order the zucchini noodles, just smile and say, "Fuck that, I'll take the carbs." Because life's too short to live without garlic bread, mashed potatoes, or a big-ass plate of spaghetti.

Fitness Lies That Need to Die: From Keto Mania to the Anti-Carb Crusade

Fitness culture loves its lies. These aren't just little white lies, like when you tell your partner their terrible cooking tastes amazing. No, these are big, ugly, gaslighting lies designed to make you hate yourself enough to throw money at detox teas, boot camps, and meal plans written by people who think iceberg lettuce is a lifestyle. It's time to drag these lies into the light and put them out of their misery, starting with the bullshit surrounding carbs and keto.

Let's kick things off with keto mania, shall we? Keto is the diet that swore up and down that you could eat bacon-wrapped butterballs for every meal as long as you avoided bread. Carbs were painted as the ultimate villain, the Lex Luthor to your Superman, the Regina George of your food pyramid. Keto promised rapid weight loss, endless energy, and the kind of abs that could slice through granite. What it didn't promise was the bad breath, mood swings, and the fact that you'd eventually want to punch anyone who said the word "ketosis" within a five-foot radius.

The problem with keto is that it's built on the same lie as every other low-carb diet: that carbs are somehow responsible for all the world's problems. Want to lose weight? Ditch the carbs. Want clear skin? Bye-bye, bread. Want to live forever? Say sayonara to spaghetti. It's all a load of horseshit, and here's why: carbs are literally your body's preferred source of energy. Cutting them out completely is like trying to run your car on vodka—it's possible, but it's going to be a bumpy fucking ride.

Keto also conveniently ignores the fact that not all carbs are created equal. Sure, eating an entire loaf of Wonder Bread in one sitting might not be the healthiest choice, but that doesn't mean all carbs are bad. Whole grains, fruits, and vegetables are packed with nutrients, fiber, and energy that your body desperately needs. Even "fun" carbs like pasta and potatoes have their place in a balanced diet. But keto doesn't care about balance. Keto cares about demonizing carbs to sell you its low-carb fantasy.

Speaking of fantasies, let's talk about the anti-carb crusade as a whole. This movement has convinced an entire generation that bread is the devil incarnate and that eating a single potato will send you spiraling into a carb-induced coma. Remember that scene in *Mean Girls* where Regina George freaks out because butter is a carb? That's the energy the anti-carb movement is working with, and it's exhausting.

One of the most infuriating lies in the anti-carb narrative is the idea that carbs make you fat. Here's the truth: eating more calories than your body burns makes you gain weight. It doesn't matter if those calories come from carbs, protein, or kale smoothies. Blaming carbs for weight gain is like blaming your shoes for your shitty dance moves—it's completely missing the point.

Another lie that needs to die is the idea that you need to "earn" your carbs. This one is especially popular in fitness culture, where people treat carbs like a reward for a hard workout. "Did you hit your macros today? Great, you can have half a sweet potato!" Fuck that. Carbs aren't a privilege—they're a basic human need. You don't have to run a marathon to deserve a bagel. You don't have to do 100 burpees to eat a slice of pizza. You're allowed to eat carbs just because you're alive and hungry, and anyone who says otherwise can fuck right off.

Then there's the lie that cutting carbs will magically make you healthier. Fitness influencers love to push this narrative, posting side-by-side photos of their "bloated" carb-eating selves and their "lean" low-carb selves. What they don't tell you is that most of that initial weight loss on a low-carb diet is just water weight. Your body stores carbs as glycogen, which holds water, so when you cut carbs, you lose water—not fat. The second you eat a slice of bread, that water comes back, and you're right where you started.

And let's not forget the low-carb product market, which is basically a giant scam. Low-carb bread, low-carb pasta, low-carb ice cream—it's all a ploy to charge you double for food that tastes half as good. Have you ever tried low-carb bread? It's like eating a sponge. Low-carb pasta? It's sadness in noodle form. Low-carb ice cream? Just eat ice cubes—it's the same experience.

The anti-carb crusade also loves to push the idea that carbs make you tired. This one kills me because carbs are literally your body's main source of energy. If you're tired after eating carbs, it's probably because you're eating a massive meal and crashing afterward—not because carbs are evil. It's like blaming your bed for making you sleepy instead of the fact that you've been awake for 36 hours.

Then there's the idea that carbs are "addictive." People love to throw around phrases like "sugar addiction" and "carb cravings" as if carbs are some kind of gateway drug. Newsflash: carbs aren't crack. They're food. Sure, we all love a warm cinnamon roll or a bowl of mac and cheese, but that doesn't mean we're addicted. It just means carbs are delicious, and anyone who says otherwise is lying to themselves.

The anti-carb narrative also conveniently ignores cultural context. For many cultures, carbs are a dietary staple. Rice, bread, pasta, tortillas— these foods have been feeding entire civilizations for centuries. The idea that these traditional, nourishing foods are "bad" is not only ignorant but also incredibly disrespectful. Imagine telling an Italian grandma that her homemade gnocchi is unhealthy. You'd get a rolling pin to the face, and honestly, you'd deserve it.

So what's the takeaway here? It's simple: carbs are not the enemy. They're not out to ruin your diet, sabotage your fitness goals, or make you fat. Carbs are fuel, joy, and tradition, and they deserve a place on your plate. The next time someone tries to sell you on keto or tells you to cut carbs, just smile, grab a bagel, and walk away. Because life is too short to live without bread, pasta, and potatoes. Fuck the lies. Eat the carbs.

"If Carbs Are Bad, Why Does Garlic Bread Taste Like a Hug from Jesus?"

Let's get one thing straight: if carbs are bad, then I don't want to be good. Because anyone who's ever had garlic bread fresh out of the oven knows it doesn't just taste good—it tastes like salvation. It's crispy, buttery, garlicky perfection, and the idea that something so divine could be "bad" is absolute fucking heresy. Fitness culture needs to sit the fuck down because there's no way I'm sacrificing breadsticks at Olive Garden for some bullshit keto bar that tastes like chalk.

This whole anti-carb narrative makes no fucking sense when you think about it. If carbs are so terrible, why do they make us feel so damn happy? Why does a big-ass plate of spaghetti feel like a warm hug on a shitty day? Why does biting into a fluffy croissant make you feel like you've ascended to another dimension? Are we really supposed to believe that the foods that bring us the most joy are somehow evil? That's like saying puppies are plotting world domination—it's absurd, and honestly, I won't stand for it.

Let's talk about bagels for a second. Bagels are fucking majestic. They're dense, chewy, and the perfect vessel for an ungodly amount of cream cheese. And yet, fitness culture wants us to believe that bagels are the dietary equivalent of committing a felony. They'll tell you to swap your bagel for a "protein-packed alternative," which is usually some sad excuse for food made out of cauliflower and broken dreams. But guess what? A cauliflower bagel is not a bagel. It's an abomination. If loving bagels is wrong, then I don't want to be right.

And don't even get me started on pasta. Pasta is the ultimate comfort food. It's versatile, satisfying, and comes in a million different forms, each more magical than the last. But fitness culture insists that we replace our fettuccine with zucchini noodles or spaghetti squash, as if that's a fair trade. Spoiler alert: it's not. Zoodles are limp, watery imposters that taste like sadness. Meanwhile, real pasta is over here living its best life, covered in creamy Alfredo or hearty Bolognese, and I'll be damned if I'm giving it up.

Speaking of substitutions, can we take a moment to acknowledge the bullshit that is "cauliflower everything"? Cauliflower rice, cauliflower pizza crust, cauliflower mashed "potatoes"—it's like fitness culture took one mediocre vegetable and decided to ruin all the good shit with it. Look, I don't have anything against cauliflower, but it's not a fucking potato, and it never will be. Stop trying to make cauliflower happen. It's not going to happen.

Then there's the absolute audacity of people who say bread is "just empty calories." Excuse me, but bread is so much more than that. Bread is history. Bread is culture. Bread is the foundation of civilizations. Jesus didn't break cauliflower with his disciples, okay? He broke bread. If it's good enough for the Last Supper, it's good enough for me.

Fitness culture also loves to guilt-trip us over pizza, as if it's some kind of dietary sin. But let's be real: pizza is the food of the gods. It's bread, cheese, and sauce—three of the greatest things in existence— combined into one glorious creation. Fitness influencers will try to tell you to make "healthier" pizza using a whole wheat crust, fat-free cheese, and some bullshit like turkey pepperoni. But that's not pizza. That's a cry for help.

And what about potatoes? Potatoes are the most versatile food on the planet. You can fry them, mash them, roast them, bake them—you name it, they're delicious. But fitness culture has turned even the humble potato into a villain. "Skip the fries," they say. "Order a side salad instead." Fuck that. Fries are crispy, salty sticks of happiness, and I'll be damned if I'm giving them up for a pile of lettuce with balsamic dressing.

The real kicker is that fitness culture never has this kind of hate for protein or fat. You never hear anyone demonizing a steak or a stick of butter. But carbs? Oh, carbs are the devil. Never mind that they're literally your body's preferred source of energy. Never mind that your brain runs on glucose, which comes from carbs. Fitness culture would rather you believe that carbs are some kind of dietary boogeyman out to ruin your life.

But here's the thing: carbs don't make you fat. Eating more calories than your body needs makes you fat. It doesn't matter if those calories come from carbs, protein, or fat—if you're eating more than you burn, you'll gain weight. Blaming carbs for weight gain is like blaming your gas pedal for a car accident. It's not the carb's fault, Karen.

The real tragedy of this anti-carb crusade is how it's robbed so many people of the simple joy of eating. Food isn't just fuel—it's pleasure, connection, and culture. It's Sunday morning pancakes with your family. It's garlic bread at a dinner party. It's pizza and beer with your friends. These moments matter, and they shouldn't come with a side of guilt.

So the next time someone tries to tell you that carbs are bad, just smile, take a big-ass bite of garlic bread, and walk away. Because if carbs are bad, then I don't want to be good. Life is too short for cauliflower rice and food guilt. Eat the bread. Order the pasta. Savor the fries. And remember: if garlic bread tastes like a hug from Jesus, then carbs are clearly on our side. Amen.

Chapter 4

Smash the Scale: Why Fitness Isn't About Numbers

The Tyranny of the Scale: Why Stepping on It Daily Is a Terrible Fucking Idea

Let's talk about the scale—that little rectangular dictator sitting smugly in your bathroom, just waiting to ruin your day. The scale is the ultimate mind-fuck, a self-esteem guillotine that can take you from "I feel amazing" to "I'm a worthless piece of shit" in 2.5 seconds. It's not a tool—it's a toxic ex-boyfriend whispering lies into your ear every morning. And yet, so many of us give it way too much fucking power.

Here's the truth about the scale: it's a lying, manipulative little asshole. It pretends to be the ultimate measure of your worth, but all it really does is show a number—a number that fluctuates depending on how much water you drank, how much salt you ate, or whether you took a dump that morning. Seriously, your weight can go up or down by five pounds in a single day, and it has absolutely nothing to do with fat. But does the scale tell you that? Nope. It just flashes its stupid little number at you and lets you spiral.

The fitness industry loves the scale because it keeps you insecure. If you're constantly chasing a lower number, you're more likely to buy into their bullshit—meal plans, supplements, gym memberships, you name it. The scale is their Trojan horse, sneaking self-doubt into your brain and convincing you that your happiness depends on reaching some arbitrary goal weight. Spoiler alert: it doesn't.

And let's not forget the emotional rollercoaster that comes with weighing yourself. Step on the scale after a week of eating clean and working out, and the number hasn't budged? Cue the self-loathing. Step on it after a weekend of pizza and beer, and it's gone up two pounds? Instant panic. The scale doesn't care about your mental health—it's there to fuck with your head and keep you second-guessing every bite of food you eat.

But the worst part about the scale is how it oversimplifies your progress. Fitness isn't just about weight—it's about strength, endurance, flexibility, and how you fucking feel. The scale doesn't measure how much stronger you've gotten, how many miles you can run, or how badass you look in those new jeans. It doesn't tell you about the muscles you're building or the energy you're gaining. It just spits out a number, and somehow, that number becomes the be-all and end-all of your self-worth.

One of the biggest lies the scale tells is that "less is better." We've been conditioned to believe that the lower the number, the more successful we are. But weight is just one tiny piece of the puzzle, and it doesn't tell the whole story. A bodybuilder and a couch potato can weigh the same, but their bodies look and function completely differently. Muscle weighs more than fat, and water weight can throw off the scale entirely. But does the scale give a fuck about context? Of course not.

The scale also doesn't account for the fact that bodies are supposed to change. Your weight fluctuates throughout your life—it's normal, natural, and not something to freak out about. You're not supposed to look the same at 40 as you did at 20. Hell, you're not supposed to look the same at 8 p.m. as you did at 8 a.m. Bodies are dynamic, and the scale doesn't reflect that.

Then there's the whole "goal weight" bullshit. Fitness culture loves to sell you the idea that happiness lies in a specific number. "If I can just get to 140 pounds, I'll feel amazing," you tell yourself. But what happens when you get there? Nothing. You're still you, with all your insecurities and hang-ups, because happiness isn't about a fucking number. It's about how you feel in your skin, and the scale has nothing to do with that.

Let's not forget the toxic rituals that come with weighing yourself. Stripping down to nothing, holding your breath, stepping on the scale like it's a firing squad, and praying for mercy. If the number goes up, you're spiraling. If it goes down, you're temporarily elated—but also terrified it'll go back up. It's a no-win situation, and honestly, who needs that kind of stress first thing in the morning?

So, what's the solution? Smash the fucking scale. Throw it out. Burn it. Give it to someone you don't like and let it ruin their life instead. You don't need a scale to tell you how you're doing. There are so many better ways to measure your progress: how your clothes fit, how much energy you have, how strong you feel, or how many stairs you can climb without wanting to puke.

Instead of focusing on the scale, focus on how you feel. Are you sleeping better? Do you have more energy? Are you kicking ass in your workouts? Those are the things that actually matter, not some arbitrary number that doesn't mean shit in the grand scheme of things.

The scale is a relic of a toxic, outdated way of thinking about fitness and health. It's time to let that shit go. You're not a number. You're a badass human being with a body that deserves love, respect, and appreciation—not judgment based on a stupid fucking rectangle. So smash the scale, and set yourself free. Because fitness isn't about numbers—it's about feeling good, living well, and giving zero fucks about what anyone else thinks.

Non-Scale Victories: How to Measure Progress Without Obsessing Over Numbers

Let's get one thing straight: the scale is not the boss of you. It's a useless little contraption that doesn't know shit about your strength, confidence, or overall badassery. The problem is, we've been brainwashed into thinking the scale is the only way to measure progress. Guess what? It's not. There are about a million other ways to know you're crushing it that have nothing to do with that lying piece of metal in your bathroom. Let's dive into the glorious world of non-scale victories (NSVs), where the wins are real, and the fucks given about numbers are zero.

First up: **your clothes.** You know that moment when you slip into a pair of jeans, and they actually fit perfectly? Like, no jumping up and down, no weird squats in the dressing room, no praying to the denim gods— just smooth sailing. That's a fucking victory. Whether your clothes are fitting better, looser, or you're finally able to zip up that jacket without feeling like a stuffed sausage, it's all a sign you're making progress. And let's be real: jeans don't lie.

Another NSV? **You're getting stronger.** Maybe you used to struggle to carry all your groceries in one trip, and now you're strutting into the house with 10 bags hanging from each arm like the Hulk. Or maybe you've gone from barely being able to do a push-up to knocking out a solid 10 like it's no big deal. That's progress, my friend. The scale might not give a fuck about your gains, but your muscles sure as hell do.

Then there's **endurance.** Remember when you used to get winded walking up a single flight of stairs? Now you're taking the stairs two at a time like you're training for the Olympics. Or maybe you've started running, and suddenly you can go a whole mile without feeling like your lungs are on fire. That's the kind of progress that actually matters—not some random number on a scale.

How about **energy levels?** If you're waking up feeling less like a zombie and more like a functional human being, that's a huge win. Or if you've got enough energy to get through your day without chugging three cups of coffee and collapsing on the couch afterward, you're doing something right. The scale can't measure how much better you're feeling, but your body sure as fuck can.

One of my personal favorite NSVs? **You're sleeping better.** Maybe you're not tossing and turning all night or waking up drenched in sweat from some stress-induced nightmare. Maybe you've even started having those deep, drooly sleeps where you wake up and have to peel your face off the pillow. That's progress, baby, and the scale doesn't have shit to say about it.

Let's talk about **confidence.** If you're starting to feel more comfortable in your own skin, that's a massive fucking win. Maybe you're rocking a crop top for the first time or strutting into the gym without giving a single fuck about who's watching. Maybe you're finally taking selfies without deleting all of them. Confidence isn't something the scale can measure, but it's a hell of a lot more important than any number.

And then there's **mental health.** If you're feeling less stressed, more focused, or just generally happier, that's a sign you're on the right track. Maybe you've started meditating, journaling, or just taking time to chill the fuck out. Whatever you're doing, if it's making you feel better, it's working.

Another underrated NSV? **Trying new shit.** Maybe you've signed up for a yoga class, joined a kickball league, or finally learned how to ride a bike without crashing into everything. The point is, you're putting yourself out there and doing things you never thought you could. That's progress, and it's fucking awesome.

Let's not forget about **relationships.** If you're feeling more present, more patient, or just generally less of an asshole to the people around you, that's a win. Maybe you've started spending more quality time with your family, or you've got the energy to actually hang out with friends instead of flaking. Whatever it is, improving your relationships is a sign that you're taking care of yourself, and that's worth celebrating.

And finally, let's talk about **happiness.** If you're laughing more, stressing less, and just generally enjoying life, that's the ultimate victory. Maybe you've started appreciating the little things, like a sunny day or a bomb-ass meal. Maybe you've stopped giving so many fucks about what other people think and started living for yourself. Whatever it is, if it's making you happy, it's progress.

The beauty of NSVs is that they're personal. They're about what matters to *you*, not what society or fitness culture says you should care about. The scale might not move, but if you're seeing and feeling these victories, you're winning in the ways that actually matter.

So fuck the scale. Celebrate the fact that you're stronger, happier, and more confident than you were yesterday. Keep smashing your goals, one badass non-scale victory at a time. Because fitness isn't about numbers—it's about how you feel, how you live, and how many fucks you don't give about the scale.

"Your Scale Is a Liar, and It Probably Hates You More Than You Hate It"

Let's talk about the scale, that smug little piece of shit lurking in your bathroom. If scales could talk, I guarantee they'd be sarcastic assholes with a voice like a cartoon villain. "Oh, you thought you were making progress? How adorable. Here, let me show you a number that'll make you cry into your protein shake." Seriously, if your scale had a personality, it would be the Regina George of fitness equipment—catty, manipulative, and thriving on your misery.

The problem with the scale isn't just that it's a liar—it's that it's a fucking *dramatic* liar. You step on it one morning, and it's like, "Congratulations, you're two pounds down!" You feel great, like you've finally got your shit together. Then, the next day, you step on it again, and it's like, "Haha, just kidding, you're three pounds up. Better cancel your plans and cry in the shower." What changed? Nothing. You drank some water, ate a salty dinner, and maybe skipped a bathroom trip. But the scale? It acts like you've single-handedly consumed the entire menu at Cheesecake Factory.

Let's not forget the emotional rollercoaster it puts you through. One second, you're on top of the world because the number went down. The next, you're questioning every life choice because it went up. And don't even get me started on those weird plateaus where the scale doesn't budge for weeks, even though you're working your ass off. It's like the scale is gaslighting you, making you feel like all your effort is for nothing.

And can we talk about how the scale has the audacity to fluctuate throughout the day? You step on it in the morning, and it gives you one number. Step on it after lunch, and suddenly it's five pounds higher. By bedtime, it's like, "Surprise, bitch! Here's a number that'll make you want to chuck me out the window." It's almost like the scale is trolling you, just waiting for the perfect moment to fuck with your head.

The real kicker is how the scale completely ignores all the important shit. Have you gained muscle? Lost inches? Improved your stamina? The scale doesn't give a fuck. All it cares about is its stupid little number, which, by the way, is affected by things like water retention, hormonal fluctuations, and whether or not you took a massive dump that morning. It's like trying to measure your self-worth with a goddamn Magic 8-Ball.

Then there's the whole ritual of stepping on the scale, which is basically a humiliation ceremony. You strip down to nothing, like taking off your socks is going to shave off an extra half-pound. You hold your breath, as if oxygen has weight. And then, you step on with the caution of someone defusing a bomb. The number flashes, and it's either the best or worst moment of your day. How the fuck did we let this little piece of plastic have so much power over us?

What's worse is how fitness culture has glorified the scale, like it's some kind of sacred oracle of truth. "Track your progress!" they say. "Weigh yourself every day!" they say. Bitch, no. Weighing yourself every day is like texting your ex—it's a guaranteed way to feel like shit for no reason. The scale doesn't measure your progress. It measures gravity's relationship with your body, and spoiler alert: gravity's kind of an asshole.

And let's not forget the times the scale decides to just completely fuck with you. You've been eating clean, working out, and feeling amazing, so you step on the scale, expecting to see some validation. But instead, it's like, "Lol, you gained four pounds." Excuse me? I've been eating kale and sweating my ass off, and this is how you repay me? Meanwhile, Karen down the street is living off wine and cheese, hasn't seen the inside of a gym in a decade, and somehow weighs less than you. Make it make sense.

The scale also loves to ruin special occasions. Got a vacation coming up? Time to stress about what the scale says before you hit the beach. Holiday season? Better freak out about every cookie you eat because the scale is watching. It's like having a toxic family member who constantly comments on your weight—except this one lives in your bathroom and never shuts the fuck up.

But here's the thing: the scale is just a tool. A shitty, outdated, overly simplistic tool that shouldn't have so much control over your life. Your worth isn't measured in pounds. Your progress isn't defined by a number. The scale doesn't know shit about your strength, your resilience, or the fact that you can now do a plank without wanting to die. It's just a hunk of plastic and metal, and it doesn't deserve the power we give it.

So what's the solution? Smash the scale. Burn it. Sacrifice it to the gods of self-love. Or, if you're not ready to go full rage mode, at least hide it somewhere you won't see it every day. Stop letting it dictate how you feel about yourself. Measure your progress in ways that actually matter: how you feel, how you move, how you live your life.

And the next time the scale tries to fuck with your head, just remember: it's a liar, a manipulator, and probably the worst roommate you've ever had. You're better than the number it spits out. You're stronger, happier, and more badass than the scale will ever acknowledge. So step off, flip it the bird, and go live your life. Because you're worth more than a stupid fucking number.

Chapter 5

Body Positivity Is for Everyone: How to Love Your Body at Every Size

Breaking Down Body Positivity: Why It's Not Just for Instagram Influencers

Let's clear something up right out of the gate: body positivity is not just for influencers with perfect lighting, strategically posed selfies, and captions that say shit like, "Love yourself, but also swipe up for my detox tea discount code." Body positivity is for everyone—yes, even you with your stretch marks, belly rolls, and that one random chin hair that grows in like it's trying to ruin your life. It's not about perfection. It's about embracing your body exactly as it is, right now, because your body is a fucking miracle, even if it feels like a pain in the ass sometimes.

Body positivity gets a bad rap because people love to twist it into something it's not. "Oh, so you're just saying we should all get fat and unhealthy?" No, Karen, that's not what I'm saying. Body positivity isn't about giving up, letting yourself go, or eating donuts for every meal (although, honestly, that sounds amazing). It's about realizing that your worth isn't tied to your weight, your size, or how well you fit into society's narrow-ass standards of beauty.

Here's the thing: society has been feeding us bullshit about our bodies for centuries. There's always some new ideal we're supposed to strive for—thigh gaps, six-packs, booty gains, cheekbones sharp enough to slice bread. And the second you get close to meeting one standard, they move the fucking goalposts. First, it was all about being thin. Then, suddenly, you needed an ass that could break the internet. Now it's abs and "strong is the new skinny." It's exhausting, and it's all designed to make you feel like you're not good enough.

But guess what? You are good enough. Right now. As you are. Body positivity is about rejecting the idea that you have to look a certain way to be worthy of love, happiness, or a decent fucking pair of jeans. It's about saying, "Fuck your beauty standards, I'm doing me."

The real beauty of body positivity is that it's not just about how you look. It's about how you *feel* in your body. Are you comfortable? Are you healthy? Are you happy? Those are the things that actually matter—not whether you have a flat stomach or a thigh gap that could double as a slip-and-slide.

Body positivity is also about recognizing that your body is more than just an ornament. It's not here to look pretty or fit into someone else's definition of hotness. Your body is your home. It's the vehicle that carries you through this messy, beautiful, chaotic life. It's your dance partner at weddings, your co-pilot on road trips, and your best fucking friend when you're lying on the couch watching Netflix. Your body is amazing, and it deserves your respect, not your criticism.

One of the biggest misconceptions about body positivity is that it's only for people who already feel good about themselves. "Oh, I could never do that," you think, as you pinch your belly or glare at your cellulite in the mirror. But that's exactly who body positivity is for. It's for anyone who's ever felt like they don't measure up. It's for anyone who's ever skipped a beach trip because they didn't want to wear a swimsuit. It's for anyone who's ever cried in a fitting room because the clothes didn't fit right.

The truth is, body positivity is a journey, not a destination. You're not going to wake up one day and suddenly love every inch of yourself. And that's okay. The goal isn't perfection—it's progress. Maybe you start by not hating yourself every time you look in the mirror. Maybe you start by wearing that outfit you've been too scared to try. Maybe you start by saying, "Fuck it, I'm eating the damn cake." Every little step counts, and every little step is a victory.

And let's be real: body positivity isn't always easy. It's hard to love your body in a world that's constantly telling you to change it. It's hard to scroll through Instagram without comparing yourself to influencers with flawless skin and abs you could do your laundry on. But the thing to remember is that those images aren't real. They're filtered, posed, and Photoshopped to within an inch of their lives. Nobody looks like that in real life—not even the influencers themselves.

The next time you catch yourself comparing your body to someone else's, take a step back and ask yourself: "Why the fuck do I care?" Their body is their business, and your body is yours. You're not in competition with anyone. You're not here to win the gold medal in hotness. You're here to live your life, love your body, and be the badass you were born to be.

Body positivity is also about appreciating what your body can do, not just how it looks. Can you walk? Dance? Hug your friends? Laugh until your stomach hurts? Those are the things that matter. Your body is capable of so much more than you give it credit for, and it's time to start celebrating that.

So let's raise a middle finger to diet culture, beauty standards, and all the bullshit that's been holding us back. Let's take up space, wear what we want, and live our lives without apology. Because body positivity isn't just for Instagram influencers. It's for all of us.

Your body is beautiful. Your body is worthy. And most importantly, your body is yours. Embrace it. Celebrate it. And love the fuck out of it.

Learning to Love Your Body: Even When It's Being a Total Pain in the Ass

Let's face it—sometimes your body is a complete asshole. It gets bloated. It breaks out. It gets sore for no fucking reason other than you slept in the wrong position. And don't even get me started on the random aches and pains that pop up as if your body is sending you a personal memo saying, "Hey, guess what? You're aging, and it's all downhill from here."

But here's the thing: your body is also your ride-or-die. It's with you for every shitty, glorious, embarrassing, and triumphant moment of your life. So, yeah, sometimes it's a pain in the ass, but learning to love it— even when it feels like it's actively plotting against you—is one of the most empowering things you can do.

Let's start with the obvious: **your body is fucking miraculous.** It keeps you alive without you having to do a damn thing. Your heart beats, your lungs breathe, your brain thinks (sometimes too much), and your digestive system does its best to process all the questionable shit you put into it. Your body is basically the MVP of your existence, and it deserves a little love for that.

That said, loving your body doesn't mean you have to be in a constant state of blissful adoration. Let's be real—nobody wakes up every day and thinks, "Wow, I look like a goddamn masterpiece." Some days you're bloated, breaking out, or just not feeling it, and that's okay. Loving your body isn't about being delusional. It's about giving it grace and appreciation, even when it's not cooperating.

For example, let's talk about those days when your body decides to be as stubborn as a toddler on a sugar high. Maybe your jeans feel tighter than they did last week, or your face is breaking out like you're 15 and stressed about prom. It's easy to fall into the trap of hating your body in these moments, but let's flip the script. Instead of focusing on the shit that's annoying you, focus on what your body *is* doing. Your legs are carrying you. Your arms are hugging the people you love. Your stomach might be bloated, but it's also digesting the tacos you had for dinner. That's a fucking win.

Learning to love your body is also about embracing the quirks—the weird, wonderful, and sometimes downright ridiculous things that make you unique. Maybe you have a scar from that time you fell off your bike as a kid, or your nose has a bump that makes it look like it's been through some shit. Those little imperfections? They're part of your story, and they're what make you *you.*

And let's not forget about stretch marks. Oh, stretch marks—the tiger stripes of life. Society tries to convince us that they're flaws, but fuck that noise. Stretch marks are proof that your body is alive, growing, and changing. They're not imperfections—they're badges of honor. So wear them proudly, like the badass you are.

Of course, loving your body also means **tuning out the bullshit.** Everywhere you look, there are ads, influencers, and self-proclaimed experts telling you how your body should look, feel, and function. "Drink this tea to flatten your stomach!" "Buy this cream to get rid of cellulite!" "Follow this workout to sculpt your abs!" It's all noise designed to make you feel like you're not enough. But here's the truth: you *are* enough, just as you are, and you don't need anyone else's validation.

One of the best ways to drown out the noise is to curate your environment. Unfollow anyone on social media who makes you feel like shit about yourself. Delete the apps that track every calorie and step like you're a goddamn lab rat. Surround yourself with people, messages, and media that lift you up instead of tearing you down. Your mental health will thank you.

Another key to loving your body is **getting comfortable with the fact that it's always changing.** Bodies aren't static. They gain weight, lose weight, stretch, shrink, sag, and wrinkle. They adapt to the seasons of life, and that's not something to fight—it's something to embrace. Your body at 20 isn't going to be the same as your body at 40, and that's not a failure. It's reality.

And let's talk about the relationship between you and your body. If you've spent years hating it, neglecting it, or punishing it, learning to love it is going to take time. You're not going to wake up tomorrow and suddenly feel like Lizzo on stage. But you can start small. Maybe it's a daily affirmation, like, "I appreciate my body for carrying me through the day." Maybe it's wearing that outfit you've been too scared to try. Maybe it's eating a meal you love without feeling guilty about it. Little by little, those small acts of kindness will add up.

One thing that helps? **Laughter.** Sometimes your body is ridiculous, and the best thing you can do is laugh about it. Got a pimple the size of a third eye? Name it. Call it Carl and joke about how it's trying to take over your life. Trip over your own feet in public? Laugh it off like you're the star of your own slapstick comedy. Your body isn't perfect, but that's what makes it human—and being human is hilarious as fuck sometimes.

Finally, remember that loving your body isn't just about how it looks. It's about how it feels, what it can do, and how it supports you every single day. It's about honoring it, respecting it, and treating it with the care it deserves. Your body is your home, your partner, and your constant companion. It might be a pain in the ass sometimes, but it's also pretty fucking amazing.

So here's to loving your body—even on the days when it feels like it's conspiring against you. Here's to celebrating the quirks, embracing the imperfections, and giving yourself the grace to just exist. Because your body is yours, and it deserves every bit of love you have to give.

"Your Body Is Like a Roommate—It's Not Always Perfect, but You're Stuck with It, So You Might as Well Make Peace"

Let's be real: your body is basically your lifetime roommate. Sometimes it's chill and helpful, like when it fights off a cold or lets you crush a workout. Other times, it's that passive-aggressive asshole who leaves dirty dishes in the sink and eats all your snacks without replacing them. But here's the thing—you can't kick your body out. You're stuck with it, so you might as well figure out how to live together without wanting to kill each other.

Think about it: your body is with you 24/7. You share everything—meals, showers, late-night Netflix binges. It hears all your secrets, feels all your emotions, and knows you better than anyone else. And yet, sometimes it acts like a total dick. Like when you wake up with a random pain in your back even though you literally did nothing except sleep. Or when your stomach decides to bloat to the size of a beach ball just because you had the audacity to eat a bagel.

But that's the deal with roommates, right? They're not always perfect. They can be annoying, messy, and unpredictable. Your body is no different. It farts at the worst possible moments, sweats through your shirt right before a big meeting, and sometimes decides to sneeze 12 times in a row just to fuck with you. But even with all its quirks and flaws, your body is still the one thing that's always there for you, no matter what.

Now, let's talk about communication. If your body were an actual roommate, you'd probably have some serious words with it on a daily basis. "Hey, body, what the fuck was that pimple doing on my chin this morning? Are we 14 again?" Or, "Really, body? You're gonna give me heartburn from eating pizza? You *loved* pizza yesterday!" The problem is, your body doesn't answer back—it just keeps doing its thing, leaving you to deal with the aftermath.

And can we talk about how your body has zero chill when it comes to aging? One day you're 25 and bouncing out of bed like a caffeinated bunny, and the next, you're 35 and making weird grunting noises every time you stand up. Your knees start cracking, your metabolism slows down, and your skin decides it's time to throw in the towel. It's like your body didn't get the memo that you're still mentally in your twenties.

But even when your body is being a total pain in the ass, it's still trying its best. Sure, it might mess up sometimes—like giving you a zit the size of Mount Everest on picture day or making you fart in yoga class—but it's also the reason you can laugh, dance, hug, and experience all the amazing things life has to offer. Your body isn't perfect, but it's yours, and that's pretty fucking cool.

Think of your body like a quirky roommate with some serious personality. Maybe it snores at night, refuses to function without coffee, and occasionally gets drunk on margaritas and makes you dance like a lunatic. But it also remembers to breathe when you forget, heals itself after you trip and fall like an idiot, and lets you experience the joy of eating tacos. It's not always easy to live with, but it's worth the effort.

And let's not forget the times your body decides to straight-up betray you. Like when your stomach suddenly rejects dairy even though you've been best friends with cheese for decades. Or when your immune system throws a temper tantrum and gives you the flu right before your vacation. It's like your body is testing your patience, daring you to lose your shit. But somehow, you make it work, because what other choice do you have?

The key to making peace with your body is learning to laugh at its ridiculousness. Got a weird mole that looks like the state of Texas?

Name it Tex and move on. Got a stretch mark shaped like a lightning bolt? Congrats, you're Harry Potter now. Your body is a treasure trove of quirks, and the more you can find humor in them, the less they'll bother you.

And let's not take for granted the times your body comes through for you like the MVP it is. Maybe it's healing that hangover after a wild night out or helping you crush a 5K you didn't think you could finish. Maybe it's letting you hug your best friend, dance like nobody's watching, or scream your lungs out at a concert. Your body is capable of so much more than you give it credit for, and it deserves some fucking gratitude.

At the end of the day, your body is your partner in crime. It's been with you through every shitty breakup, every drunken adventure, every tearful goodbye, and every laugh-until-you-can't-breathe moment. It's not perfect, but neither are you, and that's okay. Loving your body doesn't mean you have to adore every inch of it every second of the day. It just means you appreciate it for what it is—a beautifully flawed, endlessly fascinating, one-of-a-kind masterpiece.

So here's to your body, the roommate you didn't choose but couldn't live without. Here's to making peace with its quirks, laughing at its bullshit, and celebrating its awesomeness. Because at the end of the day, your body isn't just a part of you—it *is* you. And that's pretty fucking amazing.

Chapter 6

Joyful Movement: Finding Activities That Make You Happy, Not Miserable

Ditching Torture Workouts: Why You Don't Need to Punish Yourself to Stay Active

Let's start with a universal truth: working out doesn't have to feel like a fucking punishment. Somewhere along the line, fitness culture decided to sell us the idea that exercise is supposed to suck. "No pain, no gain!" they chant, as if your muscles screaming in agony is some kind of moral achievement. Bullshit. Movement should make you feel alive, not like you're auditioning for a low-budget sequel to *Saw*.

The problem is, we've been brainwashed into thinking that workouts only "count" if they're intense, miserable, and leave you in a puddle of sweat. If you're not crying on a Peloton or trying to remember your safe word at CrossFit, are you even exercising? According to fitness influencers, no. According to actual common sense, fuck yes, you are.

Let's be real: there's no glory in forcing yourself through a workout you hate. If you're dragging your ass to a boot camp at 6 a.m., cursing your life choices, and praying for a meteor to hit the building, you're doing it wrong. Exercise isn't supposed to feel like you're serving time in a maximum-security prison. It's supposed to make you feel good, both during and after. If it's not, then what's the fucking point?

Take running, for example. Some people love it. They get that "runner's high" and feel like they're gliding through life like majestic gazelles. And that's great for them. But if you hate running—like, truly despise it— stop forcing yourself to do it. Running isn't a magical key to fitness. It's just one of a million ways to move your body. If the thought of jogging makes you want to throw yourself into oncoming traffic, maybe it's time to find something else.

The same goes for spin classes, weightlifting, and every other trendy workout that's supposed to change your life. If you love them, fantastic. If you don't, fuck them. You're not a failure if you skip SoulCycle or cancel your gym membership. You're just a human being figuring out what works for you, and there's no shame in that.

The trick is to find movement that actually brings you joy. Maybe it's dancing around your living room like a drunk aunt at a wedding. Maybe it's swimming, hiking, or kayaking. Maybe it's something as simple as walking your dog or gardening. It doesn't matter what it is, as long as it makes you happy. And no, it doesn't have to "burn the most calories" or "torch fat" to be worthwhile. The goal isn't to punish your body—it's to celebrate it.

Speaking of punishment, let's talk about the absolute fuckery that is HIIT (High-Intensity Interval Training). If you love HIIT, more power to you. But for the rest of us, it feels like being trapped in a sadistic gym class where the coach has a grudge. Burpees? Fuck that. Mountain climbers? Hell no. The only "interval" I want in my life is the one between episodes of my favorite Netflix show.

And then there's the cult of CrossFit, where people willingly flip tires and climb ropes like they're auditioning for *American Gladiators*. Again, if it's your thing, go for it. But if it's not, don't let anyone guilt you into thinking you're less of a badass for skipping it. Newsflash: you can be fit without flipping a single fucking tire.

Let's also address the "calories in, calories out" crowd who treat every workout like a transaction. "Burn 500 calories to earn that slice of pizza!" they chirp, as if food is something you have to pay for with sweat. Fuck that noise. Movement isn't a punishment for eating. You don't have to "earn" your meals or "work off" dessert. Food is fuel, not a fucking bribe, and exercise is a celebration of what your body can do—not a way to atone for the sin of eating carbs.

Here's the deal: your body was made to move, but it wasn't made to suffer. The key is to find activities that make you feel good, not miserable. Maybe it's yoga, Zumba, or kickboxing. Maybe it's playing a sport you loved as a kid. Maybe it's rollerblading like it's 1995 and you're the coolest fucking person in the neighborhood. Whatever it is, if it makes you smile, you're doing it right.

And can we talk about the joy of moving for the sake of moving? Not to lose weight, not to get abs, but just because it feels good. Remember how you used to play as a kid? You ran, jumped, and climbed because it was fun, not because you were trying to hit your step count. Reclaim that joy. Dance like nobody's watching. Swing on a playground. Chase your kids around the yard. Move your body because it's fucking amazing, not because you're trying to punish it.

So here's the takeaway: ditch the torture workouts, ignore the fitness police, and find movement that makes you feel alive. Life is too short to spend it suffering through workouts you hate. Move in ways that bring you joy, make you laugh, and remind you how incredible your body really is. Because fitness isn't about pain—it's about pleasure, and you deserve every damn bit of it.

Fun Over Pain: Activities That Feel Good and Don't Make You Hate Life

Let's get one thing straight: movement doesn't have to suck. Somewhere along the way, fitness culture decided to turn exercise into a miserable grind, like it's some rite of passage to hate every second of it. "No pain, no gain," they say, like they're the gym version of a medieval torturer. Fuck that. If your workout makes you want to fake your own death to avoid it, you're doing the wrong workout.

Exercise doesn't have to be a sweaty, screaming ordeal. It can be fun. Yes, I said it—*fun*. Remember fun? That thing you used to have before adulting crushed your soul? Movement should make you feel good, not like you've been hit by a truck. So let's explore some activities that are all about pleasure, not punishment.

Dancing Like Nobody's Watching (Even If They Are)
If you're not incorporating dance into your life, you're missing out. Dancing is like flipping the middle finger to all those boring-ass workouts that feel like chores. Put on your favorite music, crank it up to an inappropriate volume, and shake your ass like you're auditioning for *Magic Mike*. It doesn't matter if you have rhythm or if your dance moves look like you're swatting at imaginary bees—just move your body and have a good fucking time.

You don't need a Zumba class or a club to dance. Your living room works just fine. And the best part? There are no rules. Twerk, shimmy, do the sprinkler—whatever makes you feel alive. Dancing isn't just exercise; it's therapy with a bass line.

Swimming: Because Gravity Is Overrated

Swimming is like a full-body workout disguised as a mini vacation. The water supports your weight, so you can move freely without feeling like your joints are plotting against you. Plus, you get to feel like a majestic sea creature, even if you're just dog-paddling across the shallow end.

Whether you're doing laps, splashing around with friends, or floating on your back like a human pool noodle, swimming is pure joy. And let's not forget the added bonus of wearing a swimsuit and not giving a single fuck about what anyone thinks. You're here to have fun, not audition for *Baywatch*.

Hiking: Nature's Gym Without the Judgy Mirrors

If you're not into the whole gym vibe, hiking is the perfect alternative. It's just you, the great outdoors, and a trail that doesn't give a shit about your insecurities. You can walk at your own pace, stop to admire the view, and maybe even take a snack break because, let's be honest, hiking snacks hit different.

The best part about hiking? It's free, it's peaceful, and it doesn't involve a single piece of gym equipment. No treadmills, no dumbbells, no overly enthusiastic trainers shouting motivational bullshit at you. Just fresh air, sunshine, and the occasional squirrel.

Rollerblading: The '90s Called, and They Said It's Still Cool

Rollerblading is the ultimate throwback activity. Strap on some skates, channel your inner '90s kid, and glide through your neighborhood like you're starring in a retro music video. It's fun, it's nostalgic, and it's a hell of a lot more exciting than running in circles at the gym.

And don't worry if you're a little rusty. Falling is half the fun. Just make sure to wear some pads so you don't end up with road rash that looks like you wrestled a porcupine. Bonus points if you blast some classic '90s jams while you skate.

Playing Sports Like You're 12 Again
Remember how much fun you had playing sports as a kid? Before everything became about winning, losing, and ruining your knees? Bring that energy back. Grab some friends, a ball, and a patch of grass, and just play. It doesn't matter if it's soccer, basketball, kickball, or even dodgeball—just find something that makes you feel like a carefree kid again.

The great thing about playing sports is that it doesn't feel like exercise. You're too busy laughing, running, and trying not to get smacked in the face with a ball to notice that you're actually working out. Plus, it's a great excuse to hang out with friends and talk shit about who's going to win.

Biking: Two Wheels and a Whole Lot of Freedom
Biking is like a ticket to your own little adventure. You can ride through the park, cruise down a quiet street, or take on a trail if you're feeling ambitious. It's low-impact, easy on the joints, and makes you feel like a kid again.

And let's be honest—there's something deeply satisfying about coasting downhill with the wind in your face. It's like flying, but without the terrifying thought of plummeting to your death. Just make sure to wear a helmet, because while biking is fun, brain injuries are not.

Yoga: Stretch, Breathe, and Pretend You're Calm

Yoga is the perfect balance of movement and relaxation. It's great for flexibility, strength, and calming the fuck down. Whether you're doing a full class or just a few poses in your living room, yoga is all about tuning into your body and appreciating what it can do.

And don't worry if you can't touch your toes or hold a pose for more than three seconds. Yoga isn't about perfection—it's about progress. So grab a mat, take a deep breath, and try not to fall over during tree pose.

Trampoline Parks: Where Gravity Goes to Die

If you've never been to a trampoline park, you're missing out on some serious fun. Jumping around like a maniac is not only a killer workout, but it's also ridiculously fun. You'll feel like a kid again—just make sure to stretch first so you don't pull a hamstring trying to do a backflip.

And let's be real—there's nothing more satisfying than launching yourself into a foam pit. It's like diving into a pool of marshmallows, but without the calories.

Ditching the Bullshit, Embracing the Fun

The bottom line? Movement doesn't have to suck. You don't need to force yourself into workouts you hate just because some influencer told you to. Find what makes you happy, and do that. Whether it's dancing, swimming, hiking, or just taking a leisurely stroll with your dog, the best workout is the one you actually enjoy.

So fuck the pain, embrace the fun, and start moving in ways that make you smile. Because life's too short for boring-ass workouts and misery-inducing gym sessions. Go out there, have fun, and let your body move the way it was meant to—with joy, laughter, and zero fucks given.

"Dancing Like Nobody's Watching Counts as Cardio—and It's Way More Fun Than a Treadmill"

Let's get this straight: cardio doesn't have to mean pounding a treadmill while staring at a clock that seems to be moving backward. Fuck that noise. Life's too short to suffer through boring workouts that make you question your existence. The truth is, cardio can be whatever the hell you want it to be, as long as it gets your heart rate up and makes you feel alive. And if it makes you laugh, even better.

Take dancing, for example. You don't need a Zumba class or a fancy studio. Just crank up your favorite playlist, channel your inner Beyoncé, and let loose. Sure, your neighbors might think you're having a seizure, but who cares? Dancing is cardio disguised as a party, and it's a hell of a lot more fun than pretending to enjoy a treadmill. Plus, where else can you twerk, do the Macarena, and attempt a TikTok dance all in one session?

If dancing isn't your thing, how about a **solo lip-sync battle?** Put on some power ballads, grab a hairbrush, and belt out your favorite songs while flailing around your living room. It's cardio and emotional therapy rolled into one. Bonus points if you include dramatic floor slides and air guitar solos. Who needs a spin class when you can sweat it out to *Bohemian Rhapsody*?

Or, let's talk about **karaoke cardio.** Gather some friends, find a karaoke machine, and sing your hearts out while jumping around like caffeinated toddlers. It's basically a workout disguised as a night out, and it burns way more calories than sitting on your ass in a bar. Plus, nothing gets your blood pumping like a spirited rendition of *Livin' on a Prayer.*

For those who need something a little less theatrical, there's always the classic **"chase the dog" workout.** Grab your furry friend, throw a ball, and spend the next 30 minutes running around like a lunatic trying to get it back. If you don't have a dog, borrow one—or better yet, just chase your cat and see how long it takes before they give you a death glare. Either way, it's cardio, and it's hilarious.

And let's not forget about the timeless appeal of **jumping on a trampoline.** It's like the universe's way of saying, "Hey, remember how much fun you used to have as a kid? Let's bring that back." Bouncing around like a maniac is a full-body workout, but it feels like pure joy. Just make sure to hold onto your dignity if you decide to try a backflip. Or don't—fuck dignity; it's overrated anyway.

If you're looking for something more adventurous, consider **"accidental parkour."** No, I'm not suggesting you leap between rooftops like a superhero, but everyday life is full of opportunities to turn regular activities into a mini obstacle course. Jump over puddles, climb onto countertops to reach that one stupidly high cabinet, or try to vault over your couch just for the hell of it. Who knew being a clumsy idiot could count as cardio?

For couples, there's always the tried-and-true option of **"sexy cardio."** You know what I'm talking about. It's the most fun you'll ever have burning calories, and it comes with the added bonus of intimacy. Just make sure you stretch first—nobody wants to explain a pulled hamstring to their doctor.

If you're feeling competitive, try **"grocery cart races."** Grab a friend, head to the store, and see who can navigate the aisles the fastest without crashing into a display of canned soup. It's cardio, comedy, and a great way to get kicked out of your local supermarket.

For those who prefer their workouts with a side of nostalgia, there's **hula hooping.** It's impossible to hula hoop without feeling like a kid again, and it's a surprisingly good core workout. Plus, it gives you an excuse to laugh at yourself when the hoop inevitably falls to the ground after two seconds.

And if all else fails, there's always **"drunk cardio."** No, I'm not saying you should chug tequila before hitting the gym, but there's something magical about drunken dance-offs and impromptu games of tag at 2 a.m. It's not the most conventional workout, but it's cardio nonetheless—and it's guaranteed to make you laugh.

The point is, cardio doesn't have to be boring or painful. It can be silly, spontaneous, and completely ridiculous. As long as you're moving, sweating, and having a good time, you're doing it right. So ditch the treadmill, grab your hairbrush, and start your own cardio revolution— because life's too short for shitty workouts and zero fun.

Chapter 7

Fuck the Fitness Police: How to Shut Down Unsolicited Opinions About Your Body

Dealing with Gym Bros and Know-It-Alls: Why Their Advice Is Unsolicited Bullshit

Let's talk about the gym bros, the Karen-level know-it-alls, and the self-proclaimed fitness experts who just *have* to share their opinions about your body and your workout routine. These are the assholes who turn the simple act of moving your body into a goddamn TED Talk you never asked for. "Oh, you're using the treadmill? You know lifting is better for fat loss, right?" Shut the fuck up, Chad.

There's a special kind of audacity that comes with offering unsolicited fitness advice. It's like these people see you at the gym, in your own lane, minding your own business, and think, "You know what this person needs? My unqualified, unwanted opinion." And don't get me started on the ones who come with that condescending tone, like they're about to grant you the secret to eternal life.

Here's the reality: 99% of the unsolicited advice you get about fitness is pure bullshit. Most of these self-proclaimed gurus are just parroting whatever they heard from some influencer on TikTok or a Reddit thread about intermittent fasting. They don't have degrees, certifications, or any actual expertise—just a massive ego and way too much free time.

And let's not forget the **gym bros**—those dudes who treat the weight rack like their personal stage. You know the ones. They grunt like they're giving birth to a fully grown rhino, drop weights as if gravity is a new concept, and constantly flex in the mirror like they're in a bad cologne ad. These guys love to swoop in with their unsolicited advice, usually while you're mid-rep and just trying to survive.

"Hey, you should really be going deeper in that squat."
"Your form is all wrong—let me show you."
"Bro, you're lifting way too light. You'll never make gains like that."

First of all, bro, *fuck off*. Nobody asked for your help. Second, if I wanted advice, I'd ask a trainer, not some dude wearing a tank top that says "Beast Mode" and smells like expired Axe body spray.

Then there are the **well-meaning Karens**—the women who think they're being helpful but are really just passive-aggressively judging you. "Oh, you're eating a protein bar? Those are so full of sugar. You should try my kale smoothie recipe instead!" No, Brenda, I don't want your fucking kale smoothie recipe. I want my chocolate-flavored bar of joy, and I don't need your commentary on my snack choices.

What makes all this unsolicited advice so infuriating is the assumption behind it: that you're not good enough as you are. That your body needs fixing, your workout needs improving, and your entire existence would be better if you just listened to them. Spoiler alert: it wouldn't.

Your body is your business, and nobody else's. Not the gym bros, not the Karens, not the influencers selling bullshit detox teas. You don't owe anyone an explanation for how you move, what you eat, or what your goals are. And you sure as fuck don't need to justify your choices to some random asshole who thinks their biceps make them a fitness authority.

So how do you deal with these fitness police without losing your shit? Let's break it down.

Step 1: The Death Stare
Sometimes, all it takes is a good old-fashioned death stare to shut someone up. Channel your inner Wednesday Addams, lock eyes with them, and let them feel the full weight of your silent, seething rage. No words necessary—just the quiet promise of destruction if they don't back the fuck off.

Step 2: The One-Liner
If the death stare doesn't work, hit them with a one-liner that makes it clear you're not here for their bullshit.
"Oh, I didn't realize you were a certified trainer. Oh wait, you're not? Cool, thanks."
"I'll take that under advisement... and then immediately ignore it."
"Wow, that's fascinating. Anyway, back to *my* workout."

Step 3: The Full-On Shutdown
For the persistent assholes who just won't quit, sometimes you need to go nuclear.

"Listen, I came here to work out, not to hear your unsolicited TED Talk on fitness. So unless you're planning to pay my membership fees, kindly fuck off."

Step 4: The Art of Ignoring

If confrontation isn't your thing, there's always the option of completely ignoring them. Put on your headphones, turn up the volume, and pretend they don't exist. Nothing says "I don't give a fuck about your opinion" like literally refusing to acknowledge their existence.

It's also worth mentioning that sometimes, the best way to deal with unsolicited advice is to laugh it off. Not because it's funny, but because it's so ridiculous that it doesn't even deserve your anger. "Oh, you think my form is wrong? Cool, thanks for your input, random stranger. Now kindly go flex in the mirror somewhere else."

And remember, you don't owe anyone a damn thing. You don't have to justify your workout, explain your goals, or even acknowledge their existence. You're at the gym (or wherever you're working out) for *you*, not to entertain their unsolicited bullshit.

At the end of the day, the fitness police are just insecure people projecting their own issues onto you. Their opinions don't matter, their advice is usually trash, and their unsolicited comments are a reflection of their own need for validation. So let them stew in their own bullshit while you focus on doing what makes you feel good.

Because the only person who gets a say in your fitness journey is you. And anyone who doesn't like that can go fuck themselves.

Reclaiming Your Space: How to Own Your Workout—or Non-Workout—Without Explanation

Let's get something straight: your body, your time, and your energy are yours. Not your trainer's, not your gym buddy's, and definitely not that random asshole at the gym who keeps trying to "fix" your form. You don't owe anyone an explanation for how you move, when you move, or if you move at all. Want to lift weights? Do it. Prefer to sit on your couch eating pizza? Fucking fantastic. Reclaiming your space means living unapologetically in your body and doing what feels right for you—no excuses, no justifications, and definitely no fucks given.

First things first: let's talk about **owning your space in the gym**. For too long, gyms have been treated like the kingdom of gym bros, where they reign supreme over the squat rack and grunt like cavemen to assert dominance. Fuck that. The gym is a shared space, and you have just as much right to be there as anyone else—whether you're bench pressing your body weight or awkwardly figuring out how the machines work.

If someone's hovering around you, waiting for you to finish your set like a vulture circling a dying animal, take your time. Stretch a little. Check your phone. Maybe even throw in an extra set just to assert your dominance. You're not on their schedule. They can wait, or they can fuck off to another machine.

And let's not forget the **mansplainers** who love to take up space in your workout, uninvited. "Hey, you know, if you adjusted your stance, you'd get a better burn." Oh, really, Chad? Did I ask for your advice? No? Then kindly go back to flexing in the mirror and leave me the fuck alone.

Reclaiming your space also means **setting boundaries with people who think your workout is a social event.** You know the type—they come over, start chatting, and before you know it, you've spent 20 minutes listening to their life story instead of actually working out. It's okay to say, "Hey, I'm here to focus on my workout, so I'll catch up with you later." Or, if you're feeling spicy, just put your headphones in mid-sentence and walk away.

And for those of you who work out at home, reclaiming your space might mean telling your family to leave you the fuck alone for 30 minutes. Put a sign on the door that says, "Do not disturb unless the house is on fire," and stick to it. Your workout time is sacred, and you deserve to have it uninterrupted—even if your dog doesn't understand why they can't sit on your yoga mat while you're in downward dog.

But reclaiming your space isn't just about the physical space—it's also about reclaiming your mental space. How many times have you skipped a workout because you were worried about looking stupid? Or tried a workout you hated because you felt like you "should"? Fuck that noise. Your workout is yours, and it doesn't have to look like anyone else's.

If you love yoga but can't touch your toes, do it anyway. If you want to dance like a maniac in your living room, go for it. If you prefer long walks to intense cardio, lace up those sneakers and strut your stuff. There's no right or wrong way to move your body, as long as it makes you feel good.

And guess what? **Not working out is also a valid choice.** Some days, the best thing you can do for your body is to give it a break. Resting doesn't make you lazy; it makes you smart. So the next time someone tries to guilt you into a workout you don't want to do, tell them, "No thanks,

I'm prioritizing my mental health today." Or, if they're really persistent, just say, "Fuck off," and go back to binge-watching your favorite show.

Reclaiming your space also means **tuning out the fitness industry's relentless guilt trips.** Everywhere you look, there are ads, influencers, and self-proclaimed gurus telling you to push harder, go longer, and never miss a workout. But guess what? You're not a fucking robot. You're a human being with needs, emotions, and a life outside the gym. You don't have to buy into the bullshit that says you're only worthy if you're constantly hustling.

Speaking of hustle culture, let's talk about the **"rise and grind" crowd—** the ones who think waking up at 4 a.m. to do burpees makes them superior. Newsflash: it doesn't. If you're not a morning person, there's no shame in sleeping in and working out later—or not at all. You're not less disciplined, less motivated, or less worthy because you value sleep over self-imposed torture.

Reclaiming your space also means **ignoring the haters.** Whether it's someone commenting on your workout (or lack thereof), criticizing your body, or making unsolicited suggestions, their opinions don't matter. You don't owe anyone an explanation for your choices, and you definitely don't owe them your time or energy.

The next time someone says, "Oh, you're doing *that* workout?" hit them with, "Yep, and I'm loving it. Thanks for your input, though." Or, if you're not in the mood for politeness, just say, "Mind your own fucking business."

Ultimately, reclaiming your space is about **taking ownership of your fitness journey—or lack thereof—and living on your terms.** It's about saying, "This is my body, my time, and my energy, and I'm going to use them in a way that feels right for me." Whether that means crushing a weightlifting session, dancing in your underwear, or skipping the workout entirely to eat ice cream in bed, it's your choice.

So own your space, unapologetically. Set boundaries, say no to unsolicited bullshit, and do what makes you feel good. Because at the end of the day, the only person you have to answer to is yourself—and you're doing just fucking fine.

"If One More Person Tells Me How to Squat, I Might Throw a Dumbbell at Their Head"

Let's talk about the unsolicited advice givers at the gym—the ones who think it's their divine mission to coach you through every single rep, whether you asked for it or not. You could be halfway through a perfectly decent squat, minding your own business, when out of nowhere, Chad from Broville decides to bless you with his wisdom. "Hey, you should go deeper in that squat. You're not engaging your glutes properly." Oh really, Chad? Thanks for the tip. Now kindly fuck off before I use this dumbbell as a projectile.

There's something uniquely irritating about the fitness know-it-all. It's like they've been waiting their whole life for this moment to shine as a self-appointed expert on human biomechanics. Never mind that they're wearing neon tank tops so tight they could double as sausage casings, or that they've been hogging the squat rack for 45 minutes doing bicep curls. Somehow, they think they're qualified to critique your form and impart their unsolicited wisdom.

And it's not just the gym bros. The fitness Karens are out there too, armed with their Pinterest quotes and green smoothies, ready to passive-aggressively comment on your workout. "Oh, you're doing squats with weights? I prefer bodyweight exercises—they're so much better for toning without bulking up." Thanks, Karen. I didn't realize I was looking for advice from someone who considers lifting their reusable water bottle a workout.

The truth is, if you're moving your body in a way that feels good for you, you're doing it right. Sure, there are some basic guidelines for not injuring yourself—like, don't try to deadlift a weight that requires a forklift—but beyond that, you don't need a fucking lecture on biomechanics from the guy who smells like stale pre-workout powder.

And let's talk about the irony of these advice givers. Half the time, their own form is so bad it looks like they're auditioning for a slapstick comedy. I once saw a guy at the gym "correct" someone's push-up form, only to go back to his bench press where he was arching his back so hard it looked like he was trying to limbo under the bar. Dude, focus on your own workout before you start handing out tips like you're the Dalai Lama of fitness.

But the unsolicited advice doesn't stop at the gym. Oh no, it follows you into every aspect of your fitness journey. Post a picture of your post-workout smoothie, and here comes someone in the comments: "You know, protein shakes are full of chemicals. You should try making your own with organic chia seeds and spirulina." Thanks, Brenda, but I think I'll stick to my store-bought sludge that tastes like chalky chocolate heaven.

Even when you're just casually talking about fitness, someone always feels the need to chime in with their two cents. "Oh, you're running? You should really switch to barefoot shoes. It's so much better for your arches." Barefoot shoes? Are you trying to ruin my life? Running is hard enough without turning it into an episode of *Survivor: Fitness Edition.*

And let's not forget the gym equipment hogs who double as fitness critics. You know the type—the ones who camp out on a machine for 20 minutes, scrolling through their phones, but still manage to find time to critique *your* workout. "Oh, you're using the leg press? You know squats are better, right?" Yes, Chad, I'm aware. But squats don't come with a built-in chair, so kindly move along.

The audacity of these people is truly something to behold. It's like they think they're doing you a favor, when really they're just making you fantasize about throwing a kettlebell through a window. And the worst part? They never seem to take the hint. You can give them the death glare, put your headphones in, and even walk away mid-sentence, and they'll still follow you like a clingy ex at a party.

But here's the thing: you don't have to listen to them. In fact, you don't owe them anything—not your time, not your attention, and definitely not an explanation for why you're doing what you're doing. Your workout is your business, and if someone doesn't like it, they can take their unsolicited advice and shove it where the sun doesn't shine.

The next time someone decides to offer their "helpful" tips, try this: "Oh, you think my form is wrong? Cool, I'll keep that in mind. Now, can you go correct someone else while I finish this set?"
Or, if you're feeling particularly spicy: "Thanks for the input, but I think

I'll stick to my routine. You can get back to yours… whenever you're done playing gym police."

And let's not forget the power of humor. Sometimes the best way to shut someone down is with a sarcastic comment that lets them know you're not here for their bullshit.
"Oh, you're an expert on squats now? That's so great for you. Maybe next you can teach me how to breathe."
"Wow, thanks for the advice, Chad. I'll be sure to add it to my collection of things I didn't ask for."

Ultimately, the key to dealing with unsolicited advice is to remember that it says more about them than it does about you. Maybe they're insecure, bored, or just really fucking annoying. Whatever the reason, it's not your problem. You're not responsible for managing their need to feel important.

So the next time someone tries to tell you how to squat, deadlift, or breathe, just smile, nod, and mentally throw a dumbbell at their head. Then go back to doing your thing, because you're crushing it—even if your form isn't textbook perfect.

At the end of the day, fitness is about moving your body in a way that feels good for you—not about pleasing the gym bros, Karens, or any other unsolicited advice givers. So own your workout, ignore the noise, and keep being the badass you are. Fuck the fitness police, and fuck their opinions. You've got this.

Chapter 8

Unfollow the Bullshit: Detoxing Your Social Media Feed from Toxic Fitness Culture

Curating a Healthier Feed: Unfollow Accounts That Make You Feel Like Shit

Let's face it: social media is a dumpster fire of unrealistic expectations, filtered abs, and influencers trying to sell you protein powder that tastes like chalk mixed with disappointment. Every time you open your feed, it's like walking into a circus of toxic fitness culture, where everyone has a six-pack, nobody sweats, and they all claim to "love" kale. Fuck that noise. It's time to detox your feed and reclaim your sanity.

Here's the thing: your social media feed should make you feel inspired, happy, or at the very least, entertained. It shouldn't make you feel like shit about yourself. If you're scrolling and suddenly thinking, "Why don't my abs look like that?" or "Maybe I *should* be drinking celery juice at 6 a.m.," it's time to hit that unfollow button like your life depends on it.

Start with the **influencers**. You know the ones. They're always posting pictures of themselves doing yoga on a beach, somehow managing to look flawless while holding a pose that would send most of us straight to the chiropractor. Their captions are filled with vague bullshit like, "Just remember: progress, not perfection," while their bodies scream, "I spend 10 hours a day working out, and I haven't eaten a carb since 2015."

Unfollow them. Seriously. If someone's account makes you feel like you're failing at life because you don't have abs that could double as a cheese grater, they don't deserve a spot in your feed. You don't need that kind of negativity, and you sure as fuck don't need their overpriced detox tea.

Next up: the **gym bros turned motivational speakers**. These are the guys who post shirtless selfies with captions like, "Pain is weakness leaving the body," or "If you're not sweating, you're not trying hard enough." Oh, really, Kyle? Is that why you're always flexing in the mirror instead of actually working out? Their entire vibe is designed to make you feel like a lazy piece of shit, but guess what? You're not lazy—you're just not a douchebag who screams at their protein shake before drinking it.

And then there's the **#Fitspiration brigade**, the ones who post quotes like, "Nothing tastes as good as skinny feels," or "Excuses don't burn calories." First of all, that's bullshit. Have these people ever tasted pizza? Ice cream? A perfectly cooked burger? Second of all, if someone's idea of motivation is shaming you into submission, they can fuck right off.

Unfollow anyone who makes you feel like your worth is tied to your weight, your workout routine, or how much you can bench press. These accounts are toxic as hell, and they don't deserve your time, attention, or Wi-Fi.

But detoxing your feed isn't just about unfollowing the assholes—it's about replacing them with accounts that actually make you feel good. Follow people who celebrate bodies of all shapes and sizes, who preach self-love without the side of shame, and who aren't afraid to admit that sometimes they skip the gym to binge-watch *Stranger Things*.

Look for accounts that make you laugh, inspire you, or remind you that fitness is about feeling good, not looking perfect. Follow people who post real shit—like their sweaty post-workout selfies, their failed attempts at yoga poses, or their honest struggles with finding motivation. These are the people who will lift you up, not tear you down.

And let's not forget about the **food porn accounts**. Follow chefs, food bloggers, and anyone who posts mouthwatering pictures of burgers, tacos, and desserts that look like they came straight out of heaven. Because here's the truth: food isn't the enemy, and you deserve to enjoy it without guilt. A feed filled with delicious-looking food is a constant reminder that life is meant to be savored—not spent obsessing over calorie counts.

Once you've detoxed your feed, you'll be amazed at how much better you feel. No more comparing yourself to impossible standards, no more guilt for skipping a workout, and no more feeling like you're not enough. Instead, your feed will be a place of positivity, humor, and inspiration—a space that celebrates you for exactly who you are.

And if you're worried about offending someone by unfollowing them, let me remind you of one important fact: your feed is *yours*. You don't owe anyone an explanation for curating it in a way that serves you. If someone's content isn't bringing you joy, hit that unfollow button and move on. It's not personal—it's self-care.

Detoxing your social media feed is one of the most empowering things you can do. It's a way of saying, "I'm done with this toxic bullshit, and I'm choosing to surround myself with positivity." So go ahead, unfollow the gym bros, the #Fitspiration queens, and anyone who tries to sell you a lifestyle that feels more like a prison sentence.

Because here's the truth: you're already enough, exactly as you are. You don't need six-pack abs, a perfect diet, or a gym membership to prove your worth. You're a badass, and no amount of filtered bullshit on Instagram can change that.

So curate your feed like your mental health depends on it—because it does. Fill it with people, messages, and content that make you smile, laugh, and feel like the incredible human you are. And when in doubt, remember this golden rule: if it makes you feel like shit, hit unfollow and never look back. Fuck toxic fitness culture, and fuck anyone who tries to tell you otherwise.

Spotting the Bullshit: How to Recognize Toxic Fitness Influencers and Their Sneaky Marketing Tactics

Let's talk about the absolute circus that is fitness influencers. These are the people who flood your social media feed with their impossibly toned bodies, perfectly lit gym selfies, and captions that sound like they were ripped from a motivational poster factory. "Be the best version of yourself!" they preach, while trying to sell you a $90 tub of "miracle" protein powder that's basically chalk dust with a fancy label. Spoiler alert: it's all bullshit.

Fitness influencers have mastered the art of sneaky marketing, and they're out here hustling like their lives depend on it. But behind every perfectly curated photo and hashtag is a pile of lies, manipulation, and outright nonsense designed to make you feel like shit about yourself so you'll buy whatever they're selling. Let's break it down, shall we?

First up: the **Before-and-After Scam**. This is one of the oldest tricks in the influencer handbook. They post a grainy, unflattering photo of themselves from "before," looking like they've just rolled out of bed after a three-day bender. Next to it, they post a glowing, high-definition photo of their "after" body, complete with abs so defined they could cut glass. "This transformation is all thanks to *SuperFit Detox Tea!*" they claim.

Yeah, sure it is. What they *don't* tell you is that the "before" photo was probably taken five minutes before the "after" photo, with bad lighting, no flexing, and a strategically bloated belly. Meanwhile, the "after" photo involves professional lighting, a flattering angle, and 20 minutes of flexing so hard they nearly passed out. It's all smoke and mirrors, folks. Don't fall for it.

Next, we have the **"Effortless Results" Lie**. This is when influencers make it seem like their flawless bodies are the result of doing three crunches a day and eating acai bowls. "You don't have to work hard to get fit!" they gush, while conveniently omitting the fact that they spend six hours a day at the gym, eat like a rabbit, and have probably had a little "help" from Photoshop—or, let's be honest, a surgeon.

And let's not forget the **"Relatable Struggle" Angle**. This is when influencers pretend to have been "just like you" before they discovered their magical fitness plan. "I used to hate my body," they say, with the kind of faux vulnerability that makes your eyes roll so hard you can see your own brain. "But then I found *ShredFit 3000,* and now I feel amazing!"

Bullshit. These people were probably born with six-pack abs and a metabolism faster than a cheetah on Red Bull. Their "relatable" story is just a marketing ploy designed to make you think, "If they can do it, so can I!" Spoiler: their results aren't from some magic plan—they're from genetics, privilege, and an unhealthy obsession with appearance.

Now, let's talk about **product endorsements**, aka the bread and butter of fitness influencers. If an influencer is holding up a product and grinning like they've just discovered the meaning of life, you can bet your ass they're getting paid to promote it. Whether it's protein powder, workout gear, or some sketchy "fat-burning" supplement, they're not selling it because it works—they're selling it because it pays.

And don't even get me started on the **detox teas and waist trainers**. These are the holy grail of fitness bullshit, peddled by influencers who swear they're the secret to their "snatched" waists. In reality, detox teas are just expensive laxatives, and waist trainers are modern-day corsets that do nothing except make it hard to breathe.

The sad truth is, influencers will slap their name on anything if the paycheck is big enough. If they're promoting something that sounds too good to be true, it probably is. "Burn fat while you sleep!" they claim, conveniently ignoring the fact that fat loss doesn't work that way and never will.

But the most insidious tactic of all is the **comparison trap**. Influencers know that if they can make you feel bad about yourself, you're more likely to buy what they're selling. So they flood your feed with pictures of their flawless bodies, their perfect diets, and their oh-so-glamorous lifestyles, all while subtly suggesting that you're not doing enough.

"Rise and grind!" they chirp, as if waking up at 4 a.m. to do burpees is the only path to success. "No excuses!" they preach, while conveniently ignoring the fact that most people don't have the time, energy, or resources to live like a fitness influencer.

Here's the kicker: most of these influencers aren't even living the life they're selling. Behind the scenes, they're just as insecure, exhausted, and human as the rest of us. They're not superhumans—they're actors in a never-ending performance of curated perfection.

So how do you spot the bullshit? Start by asking yourself a few simple questions:

- Does this influencer's content make me feel inspired, or does it make me feel like crap?

- Are they promoting a product or service that sounds too good to be true?

- Do they offer actual expertise and value, or are they just regurgitating generic motivational quotes?

If the answers don't pass the sniff test, it's time to hit that unfollow button. Your mental health is more important than following someone who makes you feel like you're not enough.

And remember, not all influencers are bad. There are plenty of fitness experts who promote healthy, realistic, and empowering messages. The key is to find the ones who align with your values and make you feel good about yourself, not worse.

At the end of the day, social media is a tool, and like any tool, it can be used for good or evil. It's up to you to curate your feed and weed out the toxic bullshit. So take back control, call out the lies, and remember: you don't need an influencer to tell you how to live your life. You're already enough, just as you are. Fuck the fitness fakes, and keep doing you.

"If Someone's Selling 'Flat Tummy Tea,' They're Not Your Friend— They're a Walking Red Flag"

Let's talk about the unholy trinity of fitness influencer scams: detox teas, miracle supplements, and waist trainers. If someone you know— or worse, someone you follow—is out here pushing "flat tummy tea" like it's the second coming of Christ, run. They're not your friend, your mentor, or your role model—they're a walking red flag with a Wi-Fi connection and no shame.

First of all, let's address the *tea* in question. It's not magic. It's not revolutionary. It's a glorified laxative in a cutesy package with a price tag that could fund a small island vacation. You're not losing weight when you drink it—you're losing the contents of your intestines at a speed that could rival a Formula 1 race car. "Flat tummy tea" isn't making you lean; it's making you dehydrated and miserable.

And yet, every influencer selling this crap wants you to believe it's the secret to their perfect body. "Just one cup a day, and you'll feel lighter and less bloated!" they chirp, conveniently leaving out the part where you'll also feel like you've been hit by a gastrointestinal hurricane. If shitting your guts out is their idea of fitness, count me the fuck out.

Now let's move on to **miracle supplements**. These are the powders, pills, and potions that promise to burn fat, build muscle, and make you look like a Greek god with zero effort. Spoiler alert: they don't work. If there were a magic pill for fitness, we'd all be popping it like Tic Tacs, and the gym industry would be out of business.

But that doesn't stop influencers from hyping this shit up like it's the holy grail. "I lost 10 pounds in two weeks thanks to *ShredFit UltraMax!*" they claim, conveniently forgetting to mention the hours they spend working out, the personal chefs preparing their meals, and the Photoshop app on their phone.

Here's a funny observation for you: if someone's selling a supplement with a name that sounds like a superhero or a video game, it's probably bullshit. "ThermoBlast Extreme?" Sounds like something that should power a rocket, not fuel your morning workout. "MegaBurn 5000?" More like MegaWasteOfMoney 5000.

And then there are the **waist trainers**, aka modern-day torture devices disguised as fitness tools. These contraptions promise to "cinch your waist" and "enhance your curves," but all they really do is squish your organs into unnatural positions and make it hard to breathe. If your workout gear makes you feel like a Victorian woman fainting on a chaise lounge, it's time to reevaluate your life choices.

The funniest part? Waist trainer influencers always post these overly enthusiastic captions like, "I love how snatched my waist looks after just one week of wearing this!" Girl, your waist looks snatched because your ribs are suffocating your spleen. That's not fitness—that's medieval cosplay.

Speaking of cosplay, let's not forget the **"fitfluencers" who hawk their own workout programs**. You know the ones. They're always posting videos of themselves doing exercises with names like "booty blasters" and "core crushers," wearing outfits so tight you wonder if they're made of body paint. "Buy my 30-day shred program for just $99.99!" they shout, as if they've cracked the code on fitness.

Newsflash: most of these programs are just generic workouts you could find on YouTube for free. The only thing "custom" about them is the poorly designed PDF they slapped their name on. Save your money and do some squats in your living room—it's just as effective, and you won't have to deal with their incessant upselling.

And let's not forget the **"holistic" influencers pushing detoxes and cleanses**. They'll have you believe that your body is a toxic wasteland in desperate need of their overpriced juices. "Rid your body of toxins!" they declare, as if your liver and kidneys aren't already doing that for free.

Here's a pro tip: if someone uses the word "toxins" without being able to explain what those toxins are, they're full of shit. Your body doesn't need a cleanse—it needs you to stop drinking $12 green sludge that tastes like lawn clippings and sadness.

Now, let's address the **social media comments section red flags**. If you see someone commenting "DM me for the secret to my transformation!" on every fitness post, block them immediately. These people are either selling scams, running pyramid schemes, or just really fucking annoying. The only "secret" they're offering is how to lose money faster than a bad bet in Vegas.

Oh, and can we talk about the **"motivational" fitness memes**? You know the ones. They're always posted by people selling some kind of bullshit product, and they say things like, "Pain is weakness leaving the body" or "Excuses don't burn calories." Really, Karen? Because I'm pretty sure laughing at your meme just burned more calories than your shitty detox tea ever will.

Ultimately, the funniest thing about these influencers is how obvious their scams are once you start paying attention. The before-and-after photos with suspiciously different lighting. The miracle products that conveniently require a subscription. The workout programs that look like they were designed by a drunk toddler. It's all so transparently ridiculous, you have to laugh.

So here's the moral of the story: if someone's selling "flat tummy tea," they're not your friend. They're a walking red flag with a sales pitch. Unfollow them, block them, or just scroll past their bullshit with a laugh and a middle finger. You don't need their scams, their lies, or their overpriced nonsense. You're better than that.

And if you ever feel tempted to buy what they're selling, just remember: your body is already amazing, detox teas are just fancy laxatives, and no supplement can replace a good laugh and a slice of pizza. Fuck the fitness scams, and fuck anyone who tries to profit off your insecurities. You're a badass, and no influencer can take that away from you.

Chapter 9

Rewriting the Rules: How to Build a Relationship with Fitness That Works for You

Your Fitness, Your Way: How to Create a Movement Routine That You Don't Hate

Let's be real: the traditional fitness rules suck. They're like an overbearing ex who always told you what to wear, what to eat, and how to live your life. "Cardio every day! No pain, no gain! You have to earn your cheat meal!" Fuck that. It's time to break up with the old rules, toss them out with last week's kale smoothie, and write a new fitness playbook—one that actually works for you.

The first step to creating a movement routine you don't hate? **Stop thinking of fitness as a punishment.** Somewhere along the line, we were all brainwashed into believing that working out is a form of penance for eating "bad" foods, skipping workouts, or simply existing in a body that doesn't look like it belongs on the cover of *Men's Health*. Guess what? You're not a fucking sinner, and you don't need to atone for your food choices or your body.

Fitness isn't about earning your calories or punishing yourself for that extra slice of pizza. It's about finding joy in movement, celebrating what your body can do, and giving yourself permission to enjoy the process. If your workout feels like a prison sentence, you're doing it wrong.

Step two: **Figure out what you actually enjoy.** This might sound like common sense, but fitness culture has convinced us that there's a "right" way to work out—and if you're not lifting heavy, running marathons, or doing CrossFit, you're somehow failing. Fuck that. The only "right" way to work out is the way that makes you feel good.

Maybe you love dancing like a maniac in your living room. Maybe you feel badass swinging a kettlebell. Or maybe your ideal workout is a long walk with your dog and a playlist of guilty-pleasure pop hits. Whatever it is, embrace it. Movement doesn't have to be complicated, trendy, or Instagram-worthy—it just has to make you happy.

And if you're not sure what you like? **Experiment.** Try a little bit of everything until you find something that sticks. Sign up for that aerial yoga class you've been curious about. Go roller skating and pretend you're in a 90s rom-com. Take a boxing class and imagine you're punching your ex's face. The beauty of fitness is that there are endless options, so don't be afraid to explore.

Step three: **Forget the "all or nothing" mentality.** One of the biggest lies fitness culture tells us is that if you're not going all out, you might as well not bother. "Go hard or go home!" they shout, as if doing a 10-minute stretch session or a quick walk around the block doesn't count. Spoiler alert: it fucking counts.

Fitness isn't about perfection—it's about consistency. It's about showing up for yourself in whatever way you can, even if that means doing half a workout or skipping it altogether because you're tired, busy, or just not feeling it. The goal isn't to be perfect; it's to create a routine that works for your life, not the other way around.

Step four: **Ditch the comparison game.** Your fitness journey is yours, and it doesn't have to look like anyone else's. Just because Karen from spin class can cycle for 90 minutes without breaking a sweat doesn't mean you have to do the same. Maybe your workout is a leisurely bike ride to the nearest ice cream shop—and guess what? That's valid as fuck.

The only person you should be comparing yourself to is past you. Did you move your body today in a way that felt good? Did you show up for yourself, even if it was just a little? Then you're winning. Fuck the noise, and focus on your own path.

Step five: **Celebrate small victories.** Fitness culture loves to glorify big milestones—running a marathon, hitting a PR, losing X number of pounds. But the real magic happens in the small wins. Maybe you walked up the stairs without getting winded. Maybe you stretched for 10 minutes before bed. Maybe you just put on your workout clothes and decided, "Fuck it, that's enough for today."

Celebrate those moments, because they're just as important as the big ones. Fitness isn't about achieving some grand, ultimate goal—it's about showing up for yourself in the little ways, day after day.

Step six: **Make it fun.** Yes, I said it: fitness can be fun. It doesn't have to be a chore, a grind, or something you dread. It can be a dance party, a hike with friends, or a game of tag with your kids. It can be whatever the fuck you want it to be, as long as it makes you smile.

If your workout feels like torture, change it. Swap the treadmill for a dance class. Trade your burpees for a game of dodgeball. Ditch the weightlifting session for a paddleboarding adventure. Life is too short for shitty workouts, so find something that lights you up and go all in.

Step seven: **Listen to your body.** This might be the most important rule of all. Your body knows what it needs, so trust it. If you're tired, rest. If you're energized, move. If you're sore, stretch. And if you're craving a day on the couch with a bag of chips and a Netflix marathon? Do that too.

Fitness isn't about pushing yourself to the brink of exhaustion or ignoring your body's signals. It's about honoring your needs, respecting your limits, and finding a balance that works for you.

At the end of the day, building a relationship with fitness is about one thing: **taking back control.** It's about rejecting the bullshit rules, finding what works for you, and doing it your way. No guilt, no pressure, no fucks given.

So go ahead—rewrite the rules, create your own playbook, and make fitness a part of your life that you actually enjoy. Because when you do it on your terms, fitness isn't just something you do—it's something that makes you feel alive.

Ditching the Rulebook: Why Breaking "Fitness Rules" Is the Ultimate Act of Rebellion

Let's get one thing straight: the "fitness rulebook" is a steaming pile of bullshit. You know the one—it's filled with all those rigid, arbitrary rules about what you're supposed to do, eat, and wear in order to be "fit." No carbs after 7 p.m., never skip leg day, and always drink a gallon of water while doing burpees. Fuck. That. Noise. Who wrote this goddamn book anyway, a sadistic gym bro with too much pre-workout and a superiority complex?

Breaking these so-called rules isn't just liberating—it's a full-on act of rebellion against a system designed to make you feel like you're never good enough. So grab your metaphorical sledgehammer and let's smash this fitness rulebook into oblivion, one stupid-ass rule at a time.

Rule #1: You Have to Work Out Every Day

Who the fuck decided this was the gold standard of fitness? Let me guess: someone who has a personal chef, a nanny, and 24 hours a day to dedicate to their abs. For the rest of us mere mortals, working out every single day isn't just unrealistic—it's a recipe for burnout, resentment, and a lifelong hatred of exercise.

Here's the truth: rest days are not the enemy. In fact, they're necessary for your body to recover and your sanity to stay intact. Skipping a workout doesn't make you lazy or weak—it makes you human. So if you need a day off (or a week off, or a month off), take it. Your worth isn't measured by the number of workouts you complete—it's measured by how many fucks you give about your own well-being.

Rule #2: Cardio Is the Key to Weight Loss

Ah yes, the great cardio myth. According to the fitness rulebook, if you're not sweating your ass off on a treadmill for an hour a day, you're wasting your time. But let me tell you something: cardio is not the magical fat-burning elixir it's made out to be. Sure, it's great for your heart and overall health, but slogging away on a stationary bike while watching reruns of *Friends* isn't the only way to move your body.

Hate running? Don't fucking run. Can't stand the elliptical? Fuck it, skip it. There are a million other ways to get your body moving, and none of them require you to spend hours doing something you hate. Dancing, hiking, playing pickleball, having a wild night in the sheets—it all counts as movement, and it's a hell of a lot more fun than counting down the seconds on a treadmill.

Rule #3: Never Skip Leg Day

The most overhyped, overused rule in gym culture. Do you know what happens if you skip leg day? Nothing. Absolutely nothing. Your legs won't fall off. Your gains won't evaporate. And despite what gym bros would have you believe, skipping leg day does not make you a fitness failure.

If you don't feel like squatting, lunging, or deadlifting, then don't fucking do it. Maybe you want to work on your arms instead. Maybe you want to lie on your couch and eat chips. Both are valid choices. The fitness police aren't going to show up at your door with a warrant for your arrest because you decided to skip a workout.

Rule #4: You Have to Track Every Calorie

Tracking calories is the bane of existence for anyone who's ever tried to "get fit." According to the rulebook, if you're not meticulously logging every bite of food you eat into an app, you're doing it wrong. But here's the thing: calorie tracking is exhausting, demoralizing, and often completely unnecessary.

Your body isn't a calculator, and your relationship with food shouldn't feel like an accounting class. If you enjoy tracking your intake, great. But if the thought of weighing your broccoli makes you want to scream into the void, ditch the fucking app and listen to your body instead. Eat when you're hungry, stop when you're full, and enjoy the damn food without obsessing over the numbers.

Rule #5: Only "Clean" Foods Are Allowed

"Clean eating" is one of the most insidious phrases to ever come out of fitness culture. It implies that there's a moral hierarchy to food, with kale and quinoa at the top and burgers and fries at the bottom. Newsflash: food doesn't have morals. It's not "clean" or "dirty"—it's just food.

If you want a salad, eat a salad. If you want a greasy, cheesy slice of pizza, eat the goddamn pizza. The fitness rulebook would have you believe that indulging in "unhealthy" foods is a crime, but the only crime here is denying yourself the joy of eating something delicious. Life is too short for bland chicken and steamed broccoli, so go ahead and order dessert.

Rule #6: Progress Means Losing Weight

This is perhaps the biggest lie in the fitness rulebook: that your worth, success, and progress can all be measured by a number on the scale. Fuck that. Your body is not a math problem to be solved, and your weight is not a reflection of your value as a person.

Progress looks different for everyone. Maybe it's feeling stronger, having more energy, or finally being able to touch your toes. Maybe it's learning to love your body as it is, without trying to shrink it into submission. Whatever your progress looks like, celebrate it—because it's yours, and it's fucking awesome.

Rule #7: Always Push Yourself to the Limit

The fitness rulebook loves to glorify pain. "No pain, no gain!" they shout, as if pulling a muscle or throwing out your back is a badge of honor. But here's the truth: pain is your body's way of telling you to stop, and ignoring it is not heroic—it's fucking stupid.

You don't have to push yourself to the brink of exhaustion to prove your dedication. Resting, modifying, and listening to your body are just as important as going hard. Fitness isn't about destroying yourself—it's about building yourself up.

Breaking the fitness rules is the ultimate act of rebellion because it's a way of saying, "Fuck the noise—I'm doing this my way." It's about rejecting the guilt, shame, and pressure that fitness culture thrives on and creating a routine that makes you feel good, not miserable.

So throw out the rulebook, grab a donut, and move your body however the fuck you want. Because the only rules that matter are the ones you make for yourself—and those rules should always include having fun, being kind to yourself, and flipping the bird to anyone who says otherwise.

"If Your Fitness Plan Includes Naps, Netflix, and the Occasional Walk, Congratulations—You've Won"

Let's get something straight: not all fitness plans have to involve grueling workouts, sweaty spin classes, or kale smoothies that taste like lawn clippings. Sometimes, the best fitness plan is the one that leaves room for naps, Netflix, and the occasional stroll to the fridge for another slice of leftover pizza. And guess what? That's not just okay— it's fucking brilliant.

You see, fitness doesn't have to be an all-or-nothing grind where you're constantly chasing some mythical version of perfection. If your idea of a "workout" is lifting the remote, clicking "Next Episode," and occasionally getting up to stretch your legs, you're already miles ahead of anyone who's spending their gym time miserable and exhausted.

Let's start with the most underrated part of any fitness plan: **naps**. You've heard the phrase "rest is important," but let's be real—most fitness gurus treat rest like it's a side dish, not the main course. Fuck that. Rest isn't just important; it's fucking sacred. Naps are nature's way of saying, "Take a break, you badass human, you've earned it."

Think about it: what's more satisfying than curling up in bed after a long day of doing whatever the hell you want? Not only does a good nap recharge your body, but it also gives your brain a chance to chill the fuck out. Sleep is where the magic happens—your muscles recover, your stress levels drop, and your brain decides that maybe, just maybe, you don't need to spiral into anxiety over that awkward email you sent this morning.

And let's not forget about **Netflix**. Some people will try to tell you that watching TV isn't "productive," but those people clearly don't understand the art of a perfectly timed binge-watch. There's nothing more cathartic than losing yourself in a show where someone else's drama is way more ridiculous than your own.

Pro tip: turn your Netflix time into a stealth workout. Throw on some yoga pants (because why the fuck not?) and stretch while watching your favorite series. Or do some squats during the opening credits. Hell, you can even count walking to the kitchen for snacks as cardio. Fitness isn't about rules—it's about getting creative and finding ways to move that don't make you want to punch someone in the face.

Speaking of movement, let's talk about **the occasional walk**. There's a reason walking has been around since humans figured out how to stand on two legs—it's simple, effective, and doesn't require a gym membership or a fancy-ass Peloton. Walking is like the gateway drug of fitness. It's low-pressure, low-impact, and you can do it literally anywhere.

Feeling adventurous? Take a walk around your neighborhood and wave at your neighbors like you're in a fucking sitcom. Prefer solitude? Pop in some headphones, blast your guilty-pleasure playlist, and strut like you're walking the runway at Paris Fashion Week.

And let's not overlook the gloriousness of **snack walks**—the perfect combination of exercise and indulgence. Stroll to your favorite coffee shop, grab a latte and a pastry, and call it a fucking workout. Bonus points if you walk back home without spilling anything.

Now, let's get into the art of **doing the bare minimum** and still winning at fitness. Some days, you're just not feeling it. Maybe it's raining, or you're tired, or you've had one too many margaritas the night before. On those days, remember: the bare minimum is still more than nothing.

Stretch in bed. Do a few leg lifts while scrolling through TikTok. Hell, even taking a long, luxurious shower can count as self-care cardio if you're scrubbing vigorously enough. The point is, you don't have to move mountains every day—sometimes, moving your ass off the couch for five minutes is a victory in itself.

And if you're someone who thrives on **multitasking**, here's a genius idea: combine your workouts with the things you already love. Love wine? Do a wine bottle workout—curl that cabernet like it's a fucking dumbbell. Love video games? Play an interactive fitness game and tell yourself it's "training for the zombie apocalypse." The possibilities are endless when you stop taking fitness so goddamn seriously.

Here's another piece of funny advice: **celebrate every tiny win like you've just run a marathon.** Did you park further away from the grocery store than usual? Congrats, you've just added extra steps to your day! Did you pick up your laundry basket and carry it up the stairs? That's strength training, baby! Did you resist the urge to tell someone off when they said, "You'd look so good if you just toned up a bit"? That's emotional endurance.

The thing about fitness culture is that it tries to make you feel like nothing you do is ever enough. But the truth is, *every little thing counts.*

You don't have to crush an intense HIIT workout to be active. You don't have to track every calorie to be healthy. You just have to do what works for you, on your own terms, and give yourself a fucking break.

So here's to naps that feel like heaven, Netflix marathons that soothe your soul, and walks that remind you that fresh air is the best kind of therapy. If your fitness plan includes these things, congratulations— you've officially won. Because at the end of the day, fitness isn't about following rules or meeting impossible standards—it's about finding joy, moving your body in ways that feel good, and living your life unapologetically.

Fuck the pressure, fuck the guilt, and fuck anyone who tries to tell you otherwise. You're doing great, you're enough, and your fitness plan— whatever it looks like—is perfect for you. Keep doing you, badass.

Chapter 10

Live Your Best, Sweatiest (or Not) Life: Fitness on Your Terms

Living Unapologetically: How to Prioritize Joy, Balance, and Freedom Over Rules

Here's the truth they don't want you to know: you don't have to follow anyone's rules to live a happy, healthy, badass life. You don't need a six-pack, a strict workout regimen, or a list of foods you've sworn off like they're your ex who cheated with your best friend. Living unapologetically means flipping the bird to the rulebook, prioritizing your joy, and doing things your way—sweaty or not.

Let's start with the whole concept of **fitness "rules."** You know the ones: workout for X minutes a day, eat "clean," burn more calories than you consume, and definitely don't enjoy carbs after 7 p.m. Who the fuck came up with this nonsense? Probably someone who thought kale was exciting and had a vendetta against donuts. Here's the thing: none of those rules were made with *you* in mind. They were made to sell shit—diets, supplements, gym memberships—and keep you chasing an impossible standard.

Living unapologetically means throwing those rules out the fucking window and replacing them with ones that make you feel good. Hate running? Don't fucking run. Love chocolate cake? Eat the damn cake. Feel like skipping the gym and dancing in your kitchen instead? Crank up the music and go full Beyoncé. Your fitness, your body, your life— your fucking rules.

Joy should always come first. This might sound revolutionary, but fitness doesn't have to be miserable. In fact, it shouldn't be. If you're forcing yourself to do workouts you hate or eat food that tastes like cardboard just to fit someone else's idea of "healthy," you're missing the point. Movement and nourishment should make you feel alive, not like you're serving a prison sentence.

Find what brings you joy and lean into it. Maybe it's hiking, swimming, or trying every class at your local studio until you find the one that makes you smile. Maybe it's walking your dog or chasing your kids around the park. Maybe it's curling up with a book and a box of cookies, knowing you're living your best life because you're doing what makes you happy.

Balance is the secret sauce. Fitness culture loves to preach extremes: all or nothing, no excuses, go big or go home. But here's the thing— extremes don't work for most people, and they sure as fuck don't lead to long-term happiness. Balance, on the other hand, is where the magic happens.

Want to have a salad for lunch and pizza for dinner? Do it. Want to crush a workout one day and binge-watch Netflix the next? Go for it. Want to take a break from the gym and focus on getting enough sleep instead? Hell yes. Balance isn't about perfection—it's about giving yourself the freedom to ebb and flow, to have good days and bad days, and to honor your body and mind without guilt or pressure.

Freedom is the ultimate goal. The freedom to live your life without obsessing over calories, steps, or how many grams of protein you've eaten today. The freedom to say no to things that don't serve you and yes to things that light you up. The freedom to stop chasing someone else's definition of fitness and create your own.

Living unapologetically means embracing that freedom with both hands and not giving a single fuck about what anyone else thinks. It means showing up for yourself in whatever way feels right in the moment and knowing that you're enough, just as you are.

And let's be clear: unapologetic living doesn't mean ignoring your health or neglecting your body. It means caring for yourself in a way that feels sustainable, joyful, and authentic. It means prioritizing movement, nourishment, and rest because you *want* to, not because you feel like you *have* to.

So, how do you start living unapologetically?
First, let go of the guilt. Stop apologizing for skipping workouts, eating "unhealthy" foods, or not fitting into society's bullshit standards. You don't owe anyone an explanation for how you live your life.

Second, stop comparing yourself to others. Your journey is yours, and it's not supposed to look like anyone else's. Celebrate your progress, honor your body, and tell anyone who tries to judge you to fuck right off.

Third, prioritize what makes you happy. If a certain workout, diet, or routine isn't bringing you joy, ditch it. Life is too short to spend it doing things that make you miserable.

And finally, give yourself permission to evolve. What works for you today might not work for you tomorrow, and that's okay. Living unapologetically means staying open to change, experimenting, and finding new ways to move, eat, and live that feel good for you.

At the end of the day, living your best, sweatiest (or not) life isn't about following rules or meeting expectations. It's about owning your choices, prioritizing your well-being, and embracing the messy, imperfect, beautiful journey of being human.

So go ahead: skip the gym, eat the carbs, and dance like nobody's watching. Live unapologetically, laugh often, and remember that you're a fucking badass, no matter how you choose to move or live. Because the best fitness plan is the one that works for you—and the best life is the one you live on your own damn terms.

Owning Your Choices: Whether You Work Out or Skip It, Do It for You

Let's cut the bullshit: whether you're hitting the gym or hitting snooze, the only person who should be calling the shots is you. Not your trainer. Not Karen from accounting who won't shut up about her new CrossFit routine. And definitely not society, with its endless noise about what you *should* be doing. Your body, your life, your fucking rules. Period.

Here's the thing about fitness culture—it thrives on guilt. It's like a toxic ex that keeps texting you at 2 a.m. with "U up?" vibes but disguised as motivational quotes. "No excuses!" they shout. "You'll regret skipping this workout!" they whine. But you know what you'll really regret? Letting someone else's bullshit dictate how you live your life.

Owning your choices means reclaiming your power and telling everyone else to fuck off. It means working out because you *want* to, not because you feel like you *have* to. And it means skipping the gym guilt-free when you're tired, busy, or just not in the mood. Because spoiler alert: you don't owe anyone an explanation for how you spend your time.

Let's start with **working out on your own terms.** Maybe you love lifting weights and feeling like a badass. Maybe you're more into yoga because stretching makes you feel less like a rusty tin man. Or maybe your idea of exercise is walking to the fridge for another beer. Whatever it is, do it because it makes you feel good—not because you think it'll make someone else approve of you.

Fitness should never be about punishing yourself or proving something to anyone else. If you're dragging your ass to the gym every day because you feel like you have to "earn" your dinner or impress strangers on Instagram, you're doing it wrong. Exercise isn't a chore; it's a fucking gift to yourself. And if it doesn't feel like a gift? Skip it and go binge-watch *The Office* for the 12th time instead.

Speaking of skipping workouts, let's talk about **owning that choice too.** Society loves to make us feel like skipping a workout is some kind of moral failure. Like the fitness gods are going to strike you down with a dumbbell if you dare to prioritize sleep or a night out with friends over burpees. But guess what? That's bullshit.

Skipping a workout doesn't make you lazy, weak, or unmotivated. It makes you human. Life happens. Schedules get busy. Sometimes you just don't fucking feel like it—and that's okay. Rest days are just as important as workout days, and listening to your body is one of the best things you can do for yourself.

The key is to make your decision intentionally, not out of guilt or obligation. If you wake up and think, "I really want to move my body today," great—go crush that workout. But if you wake up and think, "I need rest more than I need squats," then for the love of all things holy, take the rest day.

Owning your choices also means **silencing the peanut gallery.** You know the ones—the gym bros who tell you you're "wasting your potential" by not deadlifting 300 pounds. The Instagram influencers who shame you for not following their bullshit detox plan. The family members who passive-aggressively comment on your eating habits.

Here's a fun fact: none of these people get a say in your life. Their opinions are about as relevant as a Myspace profile in 2024. So the next time someone tries to guilt-trip you for skipping a workout or choosing fries over salad, feel free to hit them with a big ol' "Fuck off."

And let's not forget about **making peace with imperfection.** Fitness culture loves to preach this all-or-nothing mentality, where you're either a hardcore gym rat or a couch potato with no in-between. But real life isn't black and white—it's messy, chaotic, and full of gray areas.

Maybe you work out three days a week instead of seven. Maybe you love yoga but can't stand running. Maybe you eat salads for lunch and ice cream for dinner. None of that makes you less worthy, less disciplined, or less of a badass. It makes you fucking human.

Owning your choices also means **embracing your priorities.** If fitness is a big part of your life and makes you happy, awesome—go all in. But if you'd rather spend your time doing literally anything else, that's valid too. Your worth isn't tied to how many steps you take, how many calories you burn, or how much weight you can lift.

At the end of the day, fitness is just one part of a much bigger picture. It's not the be-all, end-all of your existence, and it's certainly not worth sacrificing your happiness, sanity, or social life for. So stop treating it like a job and start treating it like a tool—a way to feel good, not a measure of your value.

And here's the best part: **owning your choices means you get to rewrite the rules.** Want to work out twice a week and call it a day? Do it. Want to skip cardio forever and just focus on lifting? Hell yeah. Want to eat dessert every night without feeling guilty? Fuck yes, pass the brownies.

There's no one-size-fits-all approach to fitness, and anyone who tells you otherwise is full of shit. The only right way to do this is your way. So stop comparing yourself to others, stop chasing someone else's goals, and start living unapologetically.

Because at the end of the day, fitness isn't about fitting into a certain size, hitting a certain weight, or following someone else's plan. It's about finding what works for you, doing it for the right reasons, and loving yourself every step of the way. Whether you work out, skip it, or do a mix of both, do it because it feels good—not because someone told you you should.

So go ahead: make your choices, own them, and tell anyone who tries to judge you to fuck right off. You're in charge of your life, your body, and your happiness—and no one else gets to have a say in that. You're a badass, and you've got this.

"If Your Best Life Involves Yoga Pants and Zero Yoga, You're Still Winning"

Let's get one thing straight: yoga pants were not invented for yoga. Sure, that's what the marketing people want you to believe, but let's be real—nobody's buying those buttery-soft, stretchy-ass pants for downward dog. Yoga pants are for lounging, grocery shopping, and pretending you're about to work out when you're really just going to Starbucks for a venti caramel macchiato with extra whipped cream. And guess what? That's perfectly fucking fine.

The beauty of yoga pants is that they're the universal symbol of "I do what I want, when I want." You don't have to step foot in a yoga studio to rock those bad boys. You could be binge-watching Netflix, inhaling a bag of chips, or scrolling through Instagram while you sit crisscross-applesauce on your couch—and you're still winning at life. Yoga pants are less about fitness and more about *fuck-it-ness.*

But let's broaden the lens here. Living your best life doesn't have to include anything society has tried to shove down your throat as "necessary" for happiness. If you want to wear athleisure every day without breaking a sweat, congrats—you're thriving. If your idea of a workout is getting up to adjust the thermostat and then sitting back down, you're still a badass. Life isn't a competition, and there's no finish line where they hand you a trophy for doing the most squats.

Let's celebrate the little things that make life glorious, starting with **lounging in activewear.** Yoga pants, sports bras, and hoodies are the ultimate trifecta of comfort and style. Who gives a flying fuck if the only thing you're actively doing in your activewear is scrolling TikTok? If it feels good and makes you happy, that's the whole damn point.

And can we talk about the **false advertising of fitness gear marketing?** Those sweaty, smiling models doing perfect squats on a mountaintop don't represent the real-life use case for workout clothes. The real MVPs are the people who wear their running shoes exclusively for running errands and their workout tanks exclusively for drinking wine on the porch.

But the humor of this whole situation isn't just about yoga pants. It's about **rejecting the idea that you have to do certain things to "earn" happiness or self-worth.** For decades, fitness culture has been selling us the lie that joy is conditional—that you have to exercise X amount, eat X way, or weigh X pounds to be truly happy. Fuck that noise. Happiness isn't something you earn; it's something you create by unapologetically doing whatever the hell makes you feel good.

If wearing yoga pants to a barbecue where you're double-fisting hot dogs and beers makes you happy, then you're doing life right. If canceling a gym membership to use that money for spa days, movie nights, or tacos fills your cup, then cheers to you, my friend. Life's too short to spend it chasing someone else's idea of success.

And let's celebrate the audacity of doing things for **fun, not fitness.** You want to paddleboard without counting it as "calorie burn?" Hell yes. You want to hike with friends and stop every 10 minutes for snacks and selfies? Fuck yes. You want to take a Zumba class just so you can laugh at how bad your coordination is? Absolutely.

The best kind of movement is the kind that doesn't feel like a chore. It's the kind that makes you forget you're even moving because you're having so much damn fun. So ditch the step counters, the calorie trackers, and the guilt. Go play, explore, and live your life like a kid on a playground—unapologetically and without overthinking.

And let's not forget the **art of skipping workouts with flair.** Skipping the gym isn't a failure; it's a celebration of knowing what your body and mind actually need. Maybe today's not a leg day—it's a nap day. Maybe you're not in the mood for Pilates but are 100% in the mood for margaritas. That's not slacking off; that's self-care, baby.

Here's a pro tip: treat your skipped workouts like a victory, not a setback. Pour yourself a drink, put your feet up, and toast to the fact that you're prioritizing your mental health over some arbitrary fitness goal. Because at the end of the day, nobody's handing out gold medals for most consecutive days at the gym.

Let's also take a moment to laugh at the **absurdity of fitness trends.** Remember when everyone was obsessed with spin classes that felt more like nightclub raves? Or when CrossFit turned into a cult where people bragged about flipping tires? Or when goat yoga became a thing because someone decided that downward dog wasn't complete without a tiny animal shitting on your back? Fitness trends come and go, but the one constant is that you don't need to participate in any of them to live your best life.

Living your best life doesn't require a Peloton, a six-pack, or a juice cleanse. It requires *you,* fully embracing what makes you happy, whether that's eating pizza in bed, skipping cardio forever, or laughing your ass off at how ridiculous burpees are.

So here's to the joy of yoga pants with zero yoga. Here's to celebrating life on your own terms, without guilt or apology. And here's to flipping off fitness culture while you pour yourself another glass of wine. Because if you're living your best life—whatever that looks like for you—you've already fucking won.

100 Tips for Telling Fitness Culture to Fuck Off and Loving Your Life

These 100 tips are your no-bullshit guide to flipping off toxic fitness culture and embracing a life filled with joy, balance, and zero guilt. Whether you're skipping workouts or rocking yoga pants for the snacks, these tips are here to remind you that fitness is on your terms. Let's go!

Tip #1

Stop apologizing for skipping workouts. The gym doesn't give a fuck, and neither should you.

Tip #2

If your workout gear doubles as pajamas, congratulations—you've mastered life.

Tip #3

Carbs aren't the enemy. Whoever said they were can go fuck themselves.

Tip #4

Sweat is optional. Joy is mandatory.

Tip #5

The only thing you need to run from is unsolicited fitness advice.

Tip #6

Skip the burpees and do whatever the fuck makes you happy.

Tip #7

Eat the damn cake. Life's too short for kale-only diets.

Tip #8

Walking to the fridge counts as cardio if you want it to.

Tip #9

Never trust anyone who tries to sell you detox tea. They're full of shit—literally.

Tip #10

Unfollow anyone who makes you feel bad about your body. Your feed, your rules.

Tip #11

Yoga pants without yoga are still a win. Own it.

Tip #12

Skip leg day? Hell yes. Skip dessert? Never.

Tip #13

The scale is a lying asshole. Don't let it fuck with your head.

Tip #14

Celebrate every tiny win, even if it's just putting on workout clothes.

Tip #15

Life is too short for shitty workouts. Find something you love or skip it entirely.

Tip #16

Fitness isn't about punishment—it's about pleasure.

Tip #17

You don't owe anyone an explanation for your food choices. Fuck the food police.

Tip #18

Rest is productive. Anyone who says otherwise can take a seat.

Tip #19

Your body is not a "before" picture. It's perfect right fucking now.

Tip #20

Burn the fitness rulebook. You don't need it.

Tip #21

Running is optional. So is everything else.

Tip #22

You don't need a six-pack to be a badass.

Tip #23

Ice cream is a perfectly acceptable dinner. No regrets.

Tip #24

Fitness is not a one-size-fits-all thing. Make it yours.

Tip #25

Skipping workouts is self-care if that's what you need.

Tip #26

Your worth isn't measured by your steps or calories burned.

Tip #27

Fitness trends come and go. Do what works for you.

Tip #28

The best workout is the one you actually enjoy.

Tip #29

Hiking counts as exercise even if you stop for snacks every five minutes.

Tip #30

You don't have to "earn" your food. Eat the fucking pizza.

Tip #31

Skip the gym and dance in your kitchen. Same thing, but more fun.

Tip #32

Burpees are bullshit. Don't let anyone tell you otherwise.

Tip #33

Self-care sometimes looks like skipping a run for a nap.

Tip #34

Your body is a badass, no matter what size it is.

Tip #35

Celebrate non-scale victories, like not throwing your scale out the window this week.

Tip #36

No workout? No problem. You're still awesome.

Tip #37

You don't need permission to live your life.

Tip #38

Eat carbs. Love carbs. Worship carbs.

Tip #39

Your workout, your pace, your fucking rules.

Tip #40

Comparison is the thief of joy. Don't let it steal yours.

Tip #41

You're not lazy—you're human. Big difference.

Tip #42

Stretching counts as a workout if you say it does.

Tip #43

Fitness is about how you feel, not how you look.

Tip #44

Unsolicited gym advice? Politely tell them to fuck off.

Tip #45

Every body is a beach body. Period.

Tip #46

Running errands in yoga pants counts as cardio.

Tip #47

Don't chase perfection. It's overrated and exhausting.

Tip #48

Sore muscles aren't a requirement for a good workout.

Tip #49

Skip workouts guilt-free. Your mental health comes first.

Tip #50

You're enough, exactly as you are.

Tip #51

Don't let the gym bros intimidate you. You're a badass.

Tip #52

Your best life might involve Netflix and snacks. That's valid as fuck.

Tip #53

Celebrate your body for what it can do, not what it looks like.

Tip #54

Skipping one workout won't ruin your progress.

Tip #55

Sweat doesn't equal success.

Tip #56

You don't need fancy gear to move your body.

Tip #57

Skipping leg day is a human right.

Tip #58

Find your joy and stick with it.

Tip #59

The gym isn't the only place to get fit.

Tip #60

Progress isn't linear. Give yourself grace.

Tip #61

Happiness isn't found in a number on the scale.

Tip #62

Eat what you want and enjoy the fuck out of it.

Tip #63

Fitness is personal. Fuck anyone who tries to tell you otherwise.

Tip #64

Your journey is yours. Own it.

Tip #65

Skipping cardio doesn't make you a failure.

Tip #66

You're not "bad" for eating dessert.

Tip #67

Fitness should enhance your life, not control it.

Tip #68

Celebrate small victories like they're big ones.

Tip #69

Your body doesn't need fixing.

Tip #70

Exercise is optional. Joy is not.

Tip #71

Don't take fitness advice from assholes.

Tip #72

Rest is part of the process.

Tip #73

Love yourself at every stage of your journey.

Tip #74

Celebrate what your body can do.

Tip #75

Do what makes you happy. Fuck the rest.

Tip #76

Fitness isn't about punishment.

Tip #77

You're not obligated to explain your choices.

Tip #78

Every step counts, even the small ones.

Tip #79

Life is too short for shitty workouts.

Tip #80

Find movement that feels good.

Tip #81

Fuck fitness rules—they're bullshit.

Tip #82

You don't owe anyone a "before" and "after."

Tip #83

Move your body because it feels good, not because you have to.

Tip #84

Celebrate food, not fear it.

Tip #85

Be kind to yourself, always.

Tip #86

Sweaty or not, you're still winning.

Tip #87

Fitness is just one part of life—not your whole life.

Tip #88

Your worth isn't tied to your workout routine.

Tip #89

Enjoy the fuck out of your favorite foods.

Tip #90

Rest is as important as movement.

Tip #91

The best fitness plan is the one that works for you.

Tip #92

You're allowed to change your mind.

Tip #93

Celebrate every damn bite of food.

Tip #94

Stop apologizing for putting yourself first.

Tip #95

Fitness should fit your life, not the other way around.

Tip #96

You don't need anyone's approval.

Tip #97

Self-love isn't selfish—it's essential.

Tip #98

Move because you want to, not because you have to.

Tip #99

Live your best life, your way.

Tip #100

Fuck fitness culture. You're amazing just as you are.

You're the Boss of Your Own Badass Life

Well, here we are—the end of the road, the final curtain, the grand fucking finale. If you've made it this far, congratulations. You've sifted through the bullshit, laughed at the absurdity of fitness culture, and maybe even flipped the bird at a few toxic rules along the way. You've embraced the fact that fitness is not a one-size-fits-all punishment but a customizable-as-fuck journey meant to fit *your* life—not the other way around.

So what's next? Living your best, most unapologetic, sweatiest-or-not life. That means rocking yoga pants without shame (whether you're on a treadmill or on your couch). It means eating the damn carbs and not giving a single fuck about what anyone thinks. It's about saying no to burpees and yes to the activities that actually bring you joy, even if it's just walking to the freezer for ice cream.

Fitness culture will keep trying to sell you its toxic rules and guilt-trips. It'll keep whispering lies about detoxes, calorie counts, and "earning" your food. But here's the deal—you're smarter than that shit. You now know how to see through the noise, call out the bullshit, and live life on your own damn terms.

Remember, you're not in this world to make everyone else happy, to conform to someone else's standards, or to spend your precious time obsessing over a number on a fucking scale. You're here to love yourself, move your body in ways that feel good, eat food that makes you smile, and live your life in a way that makes you proud.

So go out there and be your badass self. Skip the gym if you want to, or crush a workout if that's your jam. Eat the pizza. Celebrate the little victories. Laugh at the absurdity of it all. And most importantly, never let anyone—be it Karen from spin class, your second cousin with the unsolicited advice, or some influencer selling "skinny tea"—make you feel like you're not enough.

Because you are. You're enough, exactly as you are, yoga pants, ice cream, Netflix marathons, and all. So here's to living your best life, telling fitness culture to fuck right off, and doing things your way—loud, proud, and unapologetically.

Now go be fucking amazing. You've got this.

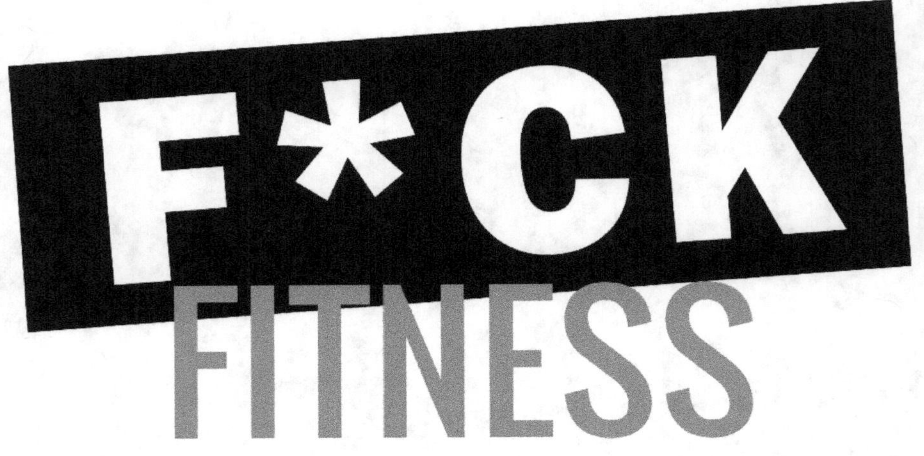

The Badass Guide to Smashing Fitness Culture One F*cking Rep at a Time!

Logan West